Official Journal of the World Psychiatric Association (WPA),

Section on Classification, Diagnostic Assessment and Nomenclature
Section on Clinical Psychopathology

Psychopathology

(Continued on next page)

Karger

Printed in Germany on acid-free and non-aging paper (ISO 9706) by Stückle Druck, Ettenheim

Karger

Printed in Germany on acid-free and non-aging paper (ISO 9706) by Stückle Druck, Ettenheim

Psychopathology

Journal Information

Aims and Scope

Psychopathology is a record of research centered on findings, concepts, and diagnostic categories of phenomenological, experimental and clinical psychopathology. Studies published are designed to improve and deepen the knowledge and understanding of the pathogenesis and nature of psychopathological symptoms and psychological dysfunctions. Furthermore, the validity of concepts applied in the neurosciences of mental functions are evaluated in order to closely bring together mind and brain. Major topics of the journal are trajectories between biological processes and psychological dysfunction that can help us better understand a subject's inner experiences and interpersonal behavior. Phenomenological and experimental psychopathology, neuropsychology and neuroscience, as well as developmental psychopathology and youth mental health contribute to this field.

Guidelines for Authors

We strongly encourage authors to read the Guidelines for Authors at www.karger.com/psp_guidelines prior to submitting an article.

Journal Contact

For questions or comments, please contact the persons responsible who can be found at http://www.karger.com/Journal/Contact/224276.

ISSN Print Edition: 0254–4962
ISSN Online Edition: 1423–033X

Journal Homepage: www.karger.com/psp
Bibliographic Indices: This journal is regularly listed in bibliographic services, including Current Contents® and PubMed/MEDLINE.

Publication Data: *Psychopathology* is published 6 times a year. Volume 53 with 6 issues appears in 2020.

Subscription Orders:
Orders can be placed at agencies, bookstores, or directly with the Publisher.

S. Karger AG
Medical and Scientific Publishers
Allschwilerstrasse 10
CH–4009 Basel
Switzerland

t: +41 61 306 11 11
f: +41 61 306 12 34
e: karger@karger.com
w: www.karger.com

(for courier services only:
Allschwilerstrasse 10
CH–4055 Basel)

Change of Address:
Both old and new addresses should be sent to the subscription source.

Subscription Rates: Subscriptions run for a full calendar year. Prices are given per year.

Personal subscription:

Print or Online	*Print+Online combined*
CHF 450.00	CHF 518.00
EUR 405.00	EUR 466.00
USD 474.00	USD 545.00

postage and handling
(added to print and print+online)
CHF 52.80 Europe, CHF 74.40 Overseas
EUR 48.00
USD 72.00

Institutional subscription:

Print or Online	*Print+Online combined*
CHF 2065.00	CHF 2375.00
EUR 1860.00	EUR 2139.00
USD 2174.00	USD 2500.00

postage and handling
(added to print and print+online)
CHF 66.00 Europe, CHF 93.00 Overseas
EUR 60.00
USD 90.00

Back Volumes and Single Issues: Information on availability and prices of single print issues and print or electronic back volumes can be obtained from Customer Service at *service@karger.com.*

Karger

Psychopathology

The Alternative Model for Personality Disorders

Guest Editor
Mark F. Lenzenweger, Binghamton, NY;
New York, NY; White Plains, NY

10 figures and 6 tables, 2020

Karger

Basel · Freiburg · Hartford · Oxford · Bangkok · Dubai · Kuala Lumpur · Melbourne · Mexico City · Moscow · New Delhi · Paris · Shanghai · Tokyo

S. Karger
Medical and Scientific Publishers
Basel · Freiburg · Hartford · Oxford ·
Bangkok · Dubai · Kuala Lumpur ·
Melbourne · Mexico City ·
Moscow · New Delhi · Paris ·
Shanghai · Tokyo

Printed on acid-free and non-aging paper (ISO 9706)
ISBN 978–3–318–06792–7
e-ISBN 978–3–318–06793–4

karger@karger.com
www.karger.com/psp

Karger

Psychopathology

Vol. 53, No. 3–4, 2020

Contents

karger@karger.com
www.karger.com/psp

Karger

Review Articles

Editorial

Psychopathology

Psychopathology 2020;53:123–125
DOI: 10.1159/000510104

Received: July 10, 2020
Accepted: July 13, 2020
Published online: August 24, 2020

Parsing and Illuminating the Personality Pathology Domain? Considering the DSM-5 Alternative Model of Personality Disorders and the Path Forward

Mark F. Lenzenweger[a, b, c]

[a]Department of Psychology, The State University of New York at Binghamton, Binghamton, NY, USA; [b]Department of Psychiatry, Weill Cornell Medical College, New York, NY, USA; [c]Personality Disorders Institute, Weill Cornell Medical College, White Plains, NY, USA

Valid parsing of the domain of personality pathology has proven to be a challenge to modern psychopathology. For many decades psychologists and psychiatrists worked with relatively vague descriptions of disordered personality, all the while knowing that certain realms of disorder were readily apparent and likely represented clinical syndromes even if etiology and pathogenesis insights remained out of reach. For example, early observers of personality pathology could point to syndromal manifestations that went by the names psychopathy, borderline personality, narcissistic pathology, and pathological dependency. Such syndromal phenotypic manifestations represented personality configurations well outside the realm of what most would consider normality, even broadly defined. These prominent clinical syndromes highlighted the need to recognize such pathology as psychopathology and define it explicitly within available classification frameworks. They also simultaneously pointed to a territory of human behavior that clearly suggested involvement of personality, but a frontier well beyond what normal personality psychologists had taken as a research focus.

The explicit definition of personality pathology emerged first in the form of relatively clearly articulated criteria sets describing a variety of recognized personality disorders in 1980 in the American Psychiatric Association's DSM-III. Some thought of these criteria as "operational," however that was incorrect as the DSM-III was merely descriptive with no hint of genuine operationism. The personality disorders defined in the DSM-III were no sooner presented than major questions arose. How best to assess the personality disorders? Were such assessments relatively free of state-trait artifacts? What was the population prevalence of personality disorders in the general population? Are personality disorders best assessed by experienced clinicians with genuine knowledge of severe personality pathology or would self-report assessments suffice? Are personality disorders truly stable, trait-like, and relatively immutable over time as suggested by all versions of the DSM nomenclatures? At present, these questions have all largely been answered to a greater or lesser extent. The structured clinical interview remains highly regarded as the assessment method of choice in many laboratories, although the role of self-report assessments is recognized and valued as well. Personality disorder assessments do not seem unduly affected by changes in mental state (i.e., anxiety, depression). Many researchers see the clear-cut utility of having clinically experienced personnel conduct personality pathology assessments, rather than inexperienced laypersons or min-

karger@karger.com
www.karger.com/psp

Karger

Mark F. Lenzenweger
Department of Psychology, The State University of New York at Binghamton
Department of Psychology, Science IV (Room G-06)
Binghamton, NY 13902 (USA)
mlenzen@binghamton.edu

imally clinically experienced research assistants. We now understand that the population prevalence of personality pathology is approximately 10%. Finally, the major longitudinal studies of personality disorder, whether working from nonclinical or clinical samples, suggest that personality pathology is plastic and malleable across meaningful periods of time – in a manner of speaking, personality pathology is neither carved in granite nor set like plaster.

In the 40 years since the publication of the criteria sets for personality disorder in the DSM-III there remain two formidable substantive challenges in the personality pathology research domain. The two challenges are indeed related and summon up an additional (third) question. The first challenge raises the question, is personality pathology best conceptualized as dysfunction that varies continuously or quantitatively, suggesting variation by degree or amount? This discussion began nearly as soon as the DSM-III was published. Some have approached the question as one of methodological preference (e.g., in clinical psychology we view human behavior in terms of continua and we measure it accordingly; in psychiatry we seek interrelated collections of signs/symptoms that hang together and represent some form of recognizable syndromal entity and we classify accordingly). Others have argued that personality pathology, even if "diagnosed" using some cutting score or diagnostic rubric, really represents continuous variation in human adjustment/illness. An observer of the personality disorder field could readily point to numerous discussions of the "pros versus cons" of diagnosis versus continuous measurement, results from innumerable factor analytic studies suggesting that continuous dimensions underlie personality pathology features (unfortunately some proponents of factor analysis sometimes neglect to emphasize that factor analysis always finds evidence of dimensions, it is simply what it does), and interesting theoretical proposals for reducing the degree of covariation seen among the well-defined domains of personality pathology (a factor complicating these discussions is that many personality disorder datasets used for reference were collected using approaches guided by a system that specifically encouraged the diagnosis of multiple pathologies in a patient).

The second challenge that remains concerns the interface of personality pathology with what is often considered the realm or constructs of normal personality. One would reasonably think that personality pathology must have something to do with normal personality as studied by normal personality psychologists. One reason this challenge has remained difficult to resolve has been that the two domains of inquiry really did not speak to one another for decades. Personality psychologists worked in academic departments of psychology at universities focusing on nonpathological subjects and personality pathologists work in psychopathology laboratories, clinics, and hospitals focusing on deeply impaired subjects. Over time the discourse between these two different worlds has increased and rich advances in our understanding of this interface have slowly emerged. The normal personality psychologist has benefitted from interaction with psychopathologists just as psychopathologists have benefitted from exposure to normal personality psychologists. This has not been a trivial development as bringing these two worlds together has allowed both to be enriched. It is the rare normal personality psychologist that fully understands the depth of impairment, the level of dysfunction, and the severity of distress found in the personality disordered patient. Psychopathologists have also been able to expand their vistas by considering a wide range of normal, healthy outcomes seen in so much of the population. Thus, the interface of personality and personality pathology is now an active area of inquiry, informed by both personality science, psychopathology, and, more recently, personality neuroscience.

The additional (third) question that emerged from the joint consideration of measurement/conceptualization concerns as well as the need to specify precise relationship among normal personality constructs and pathological personality manifestations pushes the field to consider ways in which a more unified model that can point to systems, processes, and/or dimensions that underlie the *full* range of human behavior, bridging the normal and pathological realms. Fortunately, advances made over the last 25 years have allowed for proposals that address the two main concerns raised here as well as this third derivative theoretical issue. One proposal, which embraces these foci and is now receiving careful discussion, is that found in the DSM-5 (Section III) and referred to as the Alternative Model of Personality Disorders (AMPD). The papers making up this special issue of *Psychopathology* take a careful look at the AMPD as a proposal, as a heuristic if one likes. In doing so, this array of senior researchers present, discuss, critique, and challenge the AMPD. As any long-term observer of psychopathology science, psychology, and psychiatry knows, many ideas, models, and proposals come and go in the intellectual firmament of the field. Some proposals take root and grow, whereas some proposals that generate considerable interest initially, command attention, and fill scholarly journals have been known to fade into scientific oblivion in time. This special issue places the AMPD into the academic arena for the readers of *Psychopathology*. The AMPD is a rich and challenging proposal that embodies many important assumptions, such as those discussed in this series of papers. What does the AMPD offer the field as an approach to parsing the personality pathology domain? Does it illuminate the personality/personality pathology interface? Does it help us understand process and mechanism, going beyond mere description? Does the AMPD offer a way to anchor personality and personality disorder in neuroscience, neurobehavioral systems, and/or genetics? The AMPD builds on decades of prior research and offers hints at the path forward for our understanding of personality pathology. What are the next steps in efforts seeking to unify how we understand both personality and personality pathology?

Review Article

Psychopathology

Psychopathology 2020;53:126–132
DOI: 10.1159/000508538

Received: November 18, 2019
Accepted: May 6, 2020
Published online: July 9, 2020

An Overview of the DSM-5 Alternative Model of Personality Disorders

Robert F. Krueger Kelsey A. Hobbs

Department of Psychology, University of Minnesota, Minneapolis, MN, USA

Keywords

DSM · Alternative model of personality disorders · Psychopathology · Classification systems

Abstract

Authoritative classification systems for psychopathology such as the DSM and ICD are shifting toward more dimensional approaches in the field of personality disorders (PDs). In this paper, we provide a brief overview of the dimensionally oriented DSM-5 alternative model of PDs (AMPD). Since its publication in 2013, the AMPD has inspired a substantial number of studies, underlining its generative influence on the field. Generally speaking, this literature illustrates both the reliability and validity of the constructs delineated in the AMPD. The literature also illustrates empirical challenges to the conceptual clarity of the AMPD, such as evidence of substantial correlations between indices of personality functioning (criterion A in the AMPD) and maladaptive personality traits (criterion B in the AMPD). Key future directions pertain to linking the AMPD literature with applied efforts to improve the lives of persons who suffer from PDs, and surmounting challenges germane to the evolution of the DSM itself.

Introduction

With regard to psychiatric nosology, we live in quite interesting times. Prior to the neo-Kraepelinian revolution of the 1970s, psychiatric nosology was arguably somewhat of an intellectual backwater [1]. Early 20th century efforts to classify psychopathology were largely derived from the need to keep official records, as opposed to the need to delineate a conceptual model to help direct mental health assessment and intervention. Arguably, the watershed moment that brought nosology into the limelight was the publication of DSM-III in 1980.

DSM-III was innovative in a variety of ways that are generally well known, such as the introduction of structured criteria for specific mental disorder diagnoses, which represented a notable change from the narrative approach of earlier DSMs. At that time, the multiaxial system of DSM-III was seen as an innovation that would help highlight the importance of categorical personality disorders (PDs) in characterizing a clinical case. DSM-III separated PDs from other clinical disorders by placing PDs on axis II and other disorders on axis I. This was done with the intent of highlighting the importance of personality in clinical case conceptualization, as noted by the

karger@karger.com
www.karger.com/psp

Karger

Robert F. Krueger
Department of Psychology, University of Minnesota
75 East River Road
Minneapolis, MN 55455 (USA)
krueg038@umn.edu

chairman of the DSM-IV task force, Alan Frances [2]. Frances [3] subsequently noted that a shift to a more dimensional approach to PDs was inevitable; the question was not whether this would occur, but rather, when it would occur, and what dimensional approach it would incorporate.

Consistent with Frances' prescient perspective, in the post-DSM-III era, PDs became the poster child for the conceptual and practical problems that result from trying to characterize complex clinical presentations using relatively inflexible categorical rubrics. Given the multifaceted nature of human personality, problems such as comorbidity (multiple PD labels being truly applicable to the same patient) and within category heterogeneity (notable variation in key clinical features within putatively cohesive categories) were inevitable. Although these problems were well recognized prior to and during efforts to transition from DSM-IV to DSM-5 [4], solving these problems proved to be fraught with political and practical complexities that arose during the construction of DSM-5 [5]. Also, somewhat ironically from a historical perspective, DSM-5 deleted the multiaxial approach introduced in DSM-III.

The net result of this transition was that DSM-5 contains 2 approaches to conceptualizing and diagnosing PD, the model from DSM-IV reprinted, and the model developed by the DSM-5 PD workgroup, entitled the *Alternative Model of Personality Disorders (AMPD)*. In this brief overview paper, our goals are to describe the AMPD, to give the reader a general sense of the voluminous research literature that has accumulated surrounding the AMPD since its publication in 2013, and to identify what we see as some key directions at the intersection of PDs, authoritative classification systems such as the DSM, and clinical intervention.

The Content and Structure of the AMPD

In the AMPD, the general criteria for PD consist of 7 individual criteria: A–G. The first, criterion A, refers to personality functioning. In the AMPD, the sine qua non of PD is evidence that the patient encounters difficulties with personality functioning, where functioning is understood as impairment in the sense of self and corresponding impairment in interpersonal functioning [6–8]. Criterion B refers to pathological personality traits. These traits are organized around 5 broad domains, negative affectivity, detachment, antagonism, disinhibition, and psychoticism. These domains are generally well understood as maladaptive variants of the domains of the 5-factor model of normative personality structure (Five Factor Model [9]). In the AMPD, PD is defined as the combination of clinically significant problems in functioning along with ≥1 pathological trait. In addition to these 2 primary criteria, criteria C and D refer to inflexibility and stability across time, respectively. Criteria E, F, and G refer to ensuring that the PD is not better explained by "another mental disorder" (E), the effects of a substance or a medical condition (F), and to not being normative for the person's developmental stage or sociocultural environment (G).

The AMPD also recreates DSM-IV PD constructs, working within the AMPD framework. Combinations of functioning and traits are used to recreate antisocial, avoidant, borderline, narcissistic, obsessive-compulsive, and schizotypal PD, where the target for these reconstructions was the DSM-IV descriptions of these PDs. The intent was to show how specific DSM-IV PD types could be understood as specific combinations of personality functioning and pathological traits, as opposed to categorical symptom lists. Finally, PD not otherwise specified (PD-NOS, a common DSM-IV diagnosis [10]) is replaced in the AMPD by the concept of PD trait specified. Similar to PD-NOS, the idea of PD trait specified is to capture presentations that do not fit neatly into specified types. PD trait specified allows the clinician to describe the PD in terms of a specified pattern of functioning and traits. The main difference from PD-NOS is that the clinical characteristics of the patient are specified (using concepts from the AMPD), as opposed to being "not otherwise specified," which should be advantageous in terms of clinical conceptualization and treatment selection.

The Empirical Literature on the AMPD

The AMPD has inspired a complex and vast-reaching literature, which tends to coalesce around the organization of the AMPD itself. That is, studies have tended to focus on the operationalization, reliability, and validity of criterion A and criterion B, respectively. In addition, some studies have tackled the complex issue of associations between criterion A and criterion B, in other words these studies have examined associations between functioning and traits.

The AMPD literature was reviewed very recently by Zimmerman et al. [11]. The intent of their [11] paper was to provide a comprehensive review; indeed, 318 citations are provided. Rather than duplicate this thorough, recent, and comprehensive review, here, we summarize the basic conclusions reached by Zimmermann et al. [11], organized by research on criteria A and B, and their overlap.

Criterion A: Personality Functioning

To aid the clinician in conceptualizing and assessing criterion A of the AMPD, the DSM-5 provides the Levels of Personality Functioning Scale (LPFS). Self-functioning in the LPFS is subdivided into 2 aspects, *identity* and *self-direction*. Interpersonal functioning is subdivided into 2 aspects, *empathy* and *intimacy*. Each level of each of these 4 aspects of personality functioning is described along a 5-point scale ranging from little or no impairment to extreme impairment [12, p. 775].

The LPFS has been operationalized and studied in a variety of ways, including self-report and other-report instruments, as well as structured interviews. Interestingly, interrater reliability tends to be modest but nontrivial (ICCs in the 0.4 to 0.6 range), even when raters are clinically inexperienced, and, perhaps unsurprisingly, training sessions and structured interview approaches appear to increase reported reliability coefficients [11]. This evidence is a bit surprising because the LPFS describes concepts that require some degree of psychological inference on the part of the rater (e.g., rating concepts such as a distorted self-image). Internal consistency reliability of the constructs is generally good and varies understandably by number of indicators (e.g., indices of criterion A overall, containing numerous items, tend to show higher internal consistency compared with narrower assessments containing fewer items [11]).

Regarding validity, convergent validity of criterion A measures has been documented for a variety of clinically meaningful correlates, ranging from those that are conceptually very similar (e.g., indices of PD severity from a psychodynamic perspective) to those that are more distal but still of clear clinical importance (e.g., treatment dropout [11]). Structural validity discussion in the criterion A literature tends to focus on the organizational structure described in DSM-5. That is, there is debate regarding the extent to which criterion A indices form a general dimension of personality functioning subdivided first into self and interpersonal aspects, and then further subdivided into identity and self-direction (under self) and empathy and intimacy (under interpersonal). In general, this exact proposed structure is not readily reproduced, perhaps because of the presence of a strong general factor uniting all elements of criterion A [13]. Indeed, this general PD factor may represent elements common to all psychopathology, broadly conceived (as opposed to PD specifically) [14]. In addition, performance-based assessment measures (e.g., the Social Cognition and Object Relation Scale [15]; SCORS) may provide some unique value in assessing criterion A constructs (as opposed to self-report questionnaires [16]) and should be studied more frequently in efforts to clarify the assessment and structure of criterion A.

Criterion B: Personality Traits

Criterion B of the AMPD refers to personality style and is conceptualized in terms of the 5 aforementioned trait domains of negative affectivity, detachment, antagonism, disinhibition, and psychoticism. In the AMPD, these domains are further fleshed out with 25 facets. For example, the psychoticism domain is indicated by facets labeled unusual beliefs and experiences, eccentricity, and cognitive and perceptual dysregulation.

Generally speaking, AMPD criterion B tends to be operationalized using the Personality Inventory for DSM-5 (PID-5) [17]. The PID-5 has been heavily researched; as of this writing, Google Scholar lists 1,208 citations to the paper where this measure was introduced [17]. In the self-report PID-5 literature, facet and domain scales tend to show reasonable-to-good internal consistency reliability, and the factor structure of the 25 facets tends to delineate the 5 broad trait domains listed in DSM-5 (see meta-analyses reported in Somma et al. [18] and Watters and Bagby [19]) in English and in translations of this measure [19]. There is also an extensive literature on the validity of the PID-5 showing, for example, that DSM-IV PD features can be captured by the PID-5 domains [11].

Relations between Criterion A and Criterion B

One key issue regarding the empirical evaluation of the AMPD concerns notable correlations between criterion A and criterion B constructs. These 2 elements of the AMPD reflect distinguishable traditions in PD scholarship. Criterion A reflects clinical inferences about psychological mechanisms that go awry in PD patients (pertaining to coherent conceptualization of self and other), whereas criterion B reflects the tradition of generating psychometric instruments designed to assess PD trait characteristics from the perspective of patient reports. In addition, forms of assessment other than self-report (e.g., informant and clinician reports) are applicable to both criterion A and criterion B concepts, although the literature remains tilted toward studies that rely on self-reports [11].

Empirically, at least based on the extant literature, criterion A and criterion B assessments are highly correlated, and debating the meaning of these correlations forms a key focus of the contemporary AMPD literature [11]. From our perspective, it is easy to see both sides of this debate. On the one hand, recognizing these distinguishable traditions in the PD literature by creatively synthesizing them in the AMPD represents a key opportunity for intellectual rapprochement [16]. On the other hand, the AMPD is indeed a complex model and could be considerably simplified by somehow concatenating features described in criteria A and B. These issues remain contested and are a focus of recent discussions in the literature [13, 20, 21].

Key Future Directions for the AMPD and Dimensional PD Models

Up to this point, we have focused on the AMPD of the DSM-5. In addition to the DSM, however, the other influential authoritative PD classification system is the International Classification of Diseases (ICD), published by the World Health Organization (WHO). As of this writing, the ICD-11 will become the official ICD classification system on January 1, 2022 [22]. The PD classification system that is part of the ICD-11 is a significant departure from both the previous ICD model and from categorical approaches to PD delineation [23]. Indeed, stated in terms of recent DSM models, the ICD-11 PD model is notably closer to the AMPD than to the DSM-IV PD model.

Like the AMPD, the ICD-11 PD model is dimensional, with a focus on conceptualizing PDs in terms of overall severity (akin to criterion A in the AMPD) and style (akin to criterion B in the AMPD). If a PD might be applicable to the clinical presentation, the first step is to identify the overall degree of personality difficulty on an ordinal scale (with gradations of subthreshold, mild, moderate, and severe). One option is to stop there (concluding simply that a PD is present to a specific degree) but the assessor also has the option to further describe the features of the case, using specifiers akin to the domains of the AMPD. Specifically, the ICD-11 model describes trait domains of negative affectivity, detachment, dissociality (akin to AMPD antagonism), disinhibition, and anankastia (i.e., obsessive-compulsive features). Psychoticism is omitted not because it is conceptually irrelevant to describing personality, but rather, because psychotic phenomena are described in a separate part of the ICD. The ICD-11 PD model also allows the clinician to specify a borderline pattern, to provide some continuity with classical PD constructs [24].

The ICD-11 PD model is in some ways even further of a departure from the traditional PD typological model of DSM-IV compared with the AMPD, for example. It essentially requires the diagnostician to make a dimensional (ordinal) determination of the degree of personality difficulty, in order to render any type of PD diagnosis. The general situation then, with regard to PD nosology in authoritative classification systems, entails movement toward dimensional approaches and away from classical PD categories. To our way of thinking, this makes scientific and practical clinical sense (see e.g., the discussion on clinical utility of the AMPD provided by Waugh et al. [16]). Nevertheless, the paradigm switch creates a notable disjunction with the extant PD treatment literature, and this disconnection underlines both challenges and opportunities.

Linking Developments in PD Research with Intervention Approaches

Intervention approaches for PD have historically centered around the borderline PD concept. Indeed, this is a major reason this concept was added to the ICD-11 PD model, i.e., to provide some continuity with existing approaches [23]. Comparatively less attention has been paid to the need to develop interventions applicable to other classical PDs.

There are likely numerous reasons that this situation evolved, in which the majority of treatment-oriented effort is directed at one of the 10 DSM-IV categorical PDs. Borderline PD is a very serious and debilitating condition, and efforts to intervene that are tied to this concept are to be celebrated and encouraged. Moreover, borderline PD criteria delineate the quintessence of PDs broadly conceived. From the perspective of the AMPD, borderline PD criteria emphasize difficulties in self-other conceptualization and representation (criterion A), which result in extensive manifest distress (e.g., qualities described the negative affect domain of criterion B). From this perspective, in transitioning to newer dimensional models of PD, it is critical to both recognize successes with PD intervention to date and to capitalize on opportunities to expand the armamentarium of effective prevention and intervention strategies to encompass the greater breadth of difficulties covered by AMPD criterion B. Encouraging developments along these lines can be seen in the work of Livesley et al. [25] on integrated approaches to PD treatment and Kernberg's [26] recent creative synthesis of individual differences such as temperament and intelligence with levels of personality organization that help to frame case conceptualization. Indeed, we would venture that most seasoned clinicians naturally develop multidimensional and nuanced case conceptualizations that are not readily reduced to single category labels.

The question is how to continue to pursue this progression successfully given political dynamics that naturally come into play during periods of paradigm transition. Consider, for example, some of the dynamics that have occurred in the context of the National Institute of Mental Health (NIMH)'s research domain criteria (RDoC) project. Briefly, RDoC is an effort on the part of the NIMH to encourage researchers to focus more on understanding systems that may be relevant to psychopathology (with a particular focus on neuroscience), as opposed to having their efforts constrained by thinking of classical psychiatric categories as the primary targets of empirical inquiry [27]. Pickersgill [28] recently provided a fascinating narrative account of some of the controversy in the field surrounding RDoC, in which he interviewed a series of mental health opinion leaders and summarized their perspectives and comments about RDoC. Although opinions expressed and conveyed by Pickersgill [28] were not monolithic, many are well summarized by the following quote, where "Tom" is Thomas Insel, the NIMH director who promoted RDoC during his tenure:

> I can tell you that since Tom has decided to leave nearly everyone that I've talked to has said something that they didn't feel they could say when he was still there which was that he has done more damage to clinical psychiatry than can be repaired in five or ten years [28, p 628].

Clearly, many prominent psychiatric opinion leaders reacted badly to the idea that NIMH would essentially discard cherished categorical psychiatric diagnostic rubrics in favor of the RDoC approach. Returning then to the topic of PD intervention, in the context of the AMPD, a solution may lie in viewing the multidimensional nature of case conceptualization in the AMPD framework as an opportunity to demonstrate the usefulness of a dimensional model (cf. Hopwood [29]). The acute, distressing, and life-threatening behaviors associated with borderline PD deserve the attention they have received, but also, most PD patients do not fit neatly into categorical rubrics. This leaves other characteristics (beyond those that form the understandable foci of borderline PD intervention) relatively less well conceptualized from an intervention angle. For example, emotional lability (a key criterion B facet) combined with risk taking (a separate criterion B facet that tends to vary relatively independently of emotional lability) is a different presentation from emotional lability combined with rigid perfectionism (a third criterion B facet). What is needed are case conceptualization flow charts linked to the multidimensional nature of PD variation. Reducing dimensional information to singular labels (e.g., "high on detachment") may be as problematic for reliability and case conceptualization as classical PD labels. We see the development of integrated multidimensional case conceptualization and intervention as a major opportunity in connecting developments in PD nosology with intervention efforts [30].

Evolving the DSM

Efforts by the DSM-5 PD workgroup resulted in the AMPD, which, by any standard, has been generative of extensive discussion and empirical investigation. Clearly, there is great scholarly and scientific interest in evolving PD nosologies. Interestingly, the vast majority of the AMPD literature is in psychology and not in psychiatry journals (a fact that is readily gleaned from perusing the citations given by Zimmermann et al. [11]). Perhaps this is unsurprising because psychiatry is often a conservative enterprise, for understandable reasons, such as a perceived need to preserve the tradition of the medical model as a basis for ensuring putative legitimacy. For example, it may be easier to add entirely new diagnostic categories to the DSM with only modest evidentiary support (e.g., disruptive mood dysregulation disorder [31]) than to challenge underlying assumptions (i.e., that legitimate psychiatric constructs are categorical by fiat). Other potential reasons might pertain to a preference for clinical observation as the basis for construct building (as opposed to patient reports) and the perceived clinical utility of classical category labels.

Steve Hyman, a former director of NIMH, describes this situation as "repairing a plane while it is still flying" [32]. In essence, patients and families present needing help on a daily basis and asking them to wait until we have the "perfect nosological system" is obviously impossible. From the perspective of medical authority, it is better to respond by reassuring consumers that extant approaches are valid. Nevertheless, we need to continue to provide ethical assessment and intervention, as we also strive to improve our conceptual models and corresponding intervention approaches.

From this perspective, the dynamics in play throughout the DSM-5 construction process are still active in the field. The field is slowly shifting towards more dimensional approaches to PD conceptualization. How will the DSM revision process correspond with this ongoing shift? One possibility is that the DSM continues to ossify and thereby comes to be seen as essentially irrelevant to both research and practice. Clinicians on the front lines probably do not use the DSM as intended [33], and from that perspective, the DSM being out of sync with the needs of frontline clinicians may not really constitute much of a change. Indeed, there is evidence that frontline clinicians prefer AMPD concepts (criterion B in particular) to DSM-IV PD categories in numerous respects [34]. In the research arena, the literature is now replete with concepts and approaches that are fundamentally at odds with foundational categorical assumptions of recent DSMs, such as the NIMH's dimensionally oriented RDoC project [27] and the hierarchal taxonomy of psychopathology (HiTOP) [35, 36]. Although each of these projects (the AMPD, RDoC, and HiTOP) have distinct origins and foci, they generally converge on remarkably similar broad dimensional domains for organizing the conceptualization of major individual differences relevant to psychopathology. If the American Psychiatric Association seeks to keep the DSM relevant, then the DSM will likely need to evolve along with the needs of both clinicians and researchers. Attending to these very real needs for evolution and change may be more important than seeking to promote and maintain historical psychiatric orthodoxy.

Disclosure Statement

Robert F. Krueger is a co-author of the PID-5 and provides consulting services to aid users of the PID-5 in the interpretation of test scores. PID-5 is the intellectual property of the American Psychiatric Association, and Robert F. Krueger does not receive royalties or any other compensation from publication or administration of the inventory.

Funding Sources

R.F. Krueger is supported by the US National Institutes of Health, NIH (R01AG053217, U19AG051426).

Author Contributions

R.F.K. wrote the first draft of the manuscript as an invited paper. K.A.H. provided edits to the manuscript and formatted the document. Both authors gave final approval of the completed manuscript.

References

1 Compton WM, Guze SB. The neo-Kraepelinian revolution in psychiatric diagnosis. Eur Arch Psychiatry Clin Neurosci. 1995;245(4-5):196–201.
2 Frances A. The DSM-III personality disorders section: a commentary. Am J Psychiatry. 1980 Sep;137(9):1050–4.
3 Frances A. Dimensional diagnosis of personality: not whether, but when and which. Psychol Inq. 1993 Apr;4(2):110–1.
4 Rounsaville BJ, Alarcón RD, Andrews G, Jackson JS, Kendell RE, Kendler K. Basic nomenclature issues for DSM-V. In: Kupfer DJ, First MB, Regier DA, editors. A Research Agenda for DSM-V. Washington (DC): American Psychiatric Association; 2002. pp. 1–29.
5 Zachar P, Krueger RF, Kendler KS. Personality disorder in DSM-5: an oral history. Psychol Med. 2016 Jan;46(1):1–10.
6 Morey LC, Bender DS, Skodol AE. Validating the proposed diagnostic and statistical manual of mental disorders, 5th edition, severity indicator for personality disorder. J Nerv Ment Dis. 2013 Sep;201(9):729–35.
7 Morey LC, Bender DS. Articulating a core dimension of personality pathology. In: Oldham JM, Skodol AE, Bender DS, editors. The American psychiatric publishing textbook of personality disorders. Washington, DC: American Psychiatric Association; 2014. p. 39–54.
8 Skodol AE, Morey LC, Bender DS, Oldham JM. The alternative DSM-5 model for personality disorders: a clinical application. Am J Psychiatry. 2015 Jul;172(7):606–13.
9 Widiger TA, Crego C. The Five Factor Model of personality structure: an update. World Psychiatry. 2019 Oct;18(3):271–2.
10 Verheul R, Bartak A, Widiger T. Prevalence and construct validity of Personality Disorder Not Otherwise Specified (PDNOS). J Pers Disord. 2007 Aug;21(4):359–70.
11 Zimmermann J, Kerber A, Rek K, Hopwood CJ, Krueger RF. A brief but comprehensive review of research of the alternative model for personality disorders. Curr Psychiatry Rep. 2019 Aug;21(9):92.
12 American Psychiatric Association. Diagnostic and statistical manual of mental disorders. 5th ed. Arlington (VA): American Psychiatric Association; 2013.
13 Sleep CE, Lynam DR, Widiger TA, Crowe ML, Miller JD. An evaluation of DSM-5 Section III personality disorder Criterion A (impairment) in accounting for psychopathology. Psychol Assess. 2019 Oct;31(10):1181–91.
14 Widiger TA, Bach B, Chmielewski M, Clark LA, DeYoung C, Hopwood CJ, et al. Criterion A of the AMPD in HiTOP. J Pers Assess. 2019 Jul-Aug;101(4):345–55.
15 Westen D, Lohr N, Silk KR, Gold L, Kerber K. Object relations and social cognition in borderlines, major depressives, and normals: a thematic apperception test analysis. Psychol Assess. 1990;2(4):355–64.
16 Waugh MH, Hopwood CJ, Krueger RF, Morey LC, Pincus AL, Wright AG. Psychological assessment with the DSM-5 alternative model for personality disorders: tradition and innovation. Prof Psychol Res Pr. 2017 Apr;48(2):79–89.
17 Krueger RF, Derringer J, Markon KE, Watson D, Skodol AE. Initial construction of a maladaptive personality trait model and inventory for DSM-5. Psychol Med. 2012 Sep;42(9):1879–90.
18 Somma A, Krueger RF, Markon KE, Fossati A. The replicability of the personality inventory for DSM-5 domain scale factor structure in U.S. and non-U.S. samples: A quantitative review of the published literature. Psychol Assess. 2019 Jul;31(7):861–77.
19 Watters CA, Bagby RM. A meta-analysis of the five-factor internal structure of the Personality Inventory for DSM-5. Psychol Assess. 2018 Sep;30(9):1255–60.

20 Morey LC. Thoughts on the assessment of the DSM-5 alternative model for personality disorders: comment on Sleep et al. (2019). Psychol Assess. 2019 Oct;31(10):1192–9.
21 Sleep CE, Lynam DR, Widiger TA, Crowe ML, Miller JD. Difficulties with the conceptualization and assessment of Criterion A in the DSM-5 alternative model of personality disorder: A reply to Morey (2019). Psychol Assess. 2019 Oct;31(10):1200–5.
22 World Health Organization. Eleventh revision of the International Classification of Diseases. Report by the Director-General. Executive Board 144th session, Provisional agenda item 5.9. 2018. Available from: http://apps.who.int/gb/ebwha/pdf_files/EB144/B144_22-en.pdf
23 Tyrer P, Mulder R, Kim YR, Crawford MJ. The development of the ICD-11 classification of PD: an amalgam of science, pragmatism, and politics. Annu Rev Clin Psychol. 2019 May;15:481–502.
24 Herpertz SC, Huprich SK, Bohus M, Chanen A, Goodman M, Mehlum L, et al. The challenge of transforming the diagnostic system of personality disorders. J Pers Disord. 2017 Oct;31(5):577–89.
25 Livesley WJ, Dimaggio G, Clarkin JF, editors. Integrated treatment for personality disorder: A modular approach. Guilford Publications; 2015.
26 Kernberg OF. What is Personality? J Pers Disord. 2016 Apr;30(2):145–56.
27 Kozak MJ, Cuthbert BN. The NIMH research domain criteria initiative: Background, issues, and pragmatics. Psychophysiology. 2016 Mar; 53(3):286–97.
28 Pickersgill M. Psychiatry and the Sociology of Novelty: Negotiating the US National Institute of Mental Health "Research Domain Criteria" (RDoC). Sci Technol Human Values. 2019 Jul;44(4):612–33.
29 Hopwood CJ. A framework for treating DSM-5 alternative model for personality disorder features. Personal Ment Health. 2018 May; 12(2):107–25.
30 Huprich SK. Moving beyond categories and dimensions in personality pathology assessment and diagnosis. Br J Psychiatry. 2018 Dec;213(6):685–9.
31 Evans SC, Burke JD, Roberts MC, Fite PJ, Lochman JE, de la Peña FR, et al. Irritability in child and adolescent psychopathology: an integrative review for ICD-11. Clin Psychol Rev. 2017 Apr;53:29–45.
32 Hyman SE. Diagnosing the DSM: diagnostic classification needs fundamental reform. Cerebrum. 2011 Mar;2011:6.
33 First MB, Bhat V, Adler D, Dixon L, Goldman B, Koh S, et al. How do clinicians actually use the Diagnostic and Statistical Manual of Mental Disorders in clinical practice and why we need to know more. J Nerv Ment Dis. 2014 Dec;202(12):841–4.
34 Morey LC, Skodol AE, Oldham JM. Clinician judgments of clinical utility: A comparison of DSM-IV-TR personality disorders and the alternative model for DSM-5 personality disorders. J Abnorm Psychol. 2014 May;123(2): 398–405.
35 Kotov R, Krueger RF, Watson D, Achenbach TM, Althoff RR, Bagby RM, et al. The hierarchical taxonomy of psychopathology (HiTOP): a dimensional alternative to traditional nosologies. J Abnorm Psychol. 2017 May; 126(4):454–77.
36 Krueger RF, Kotov R, Watson D, Forbes MK, Eaton NR, Ruggero CJ, et al. Progress in achieving quantitative classification of psychopathology. World Psychiatry. 2018 Oct; 17(3):282–93.

Psychopathology

Review Article

Psychopathology 2020;53:133–140
DOI: 10.1159/000506313

Received: November 21, 2019
Accepted after revision: January 31, 2020
Published online: February 28, 2020

Importance of Self and Other in Defining Personality Pathology

Aaron L. Pincus[a] Nicole M. Cain[b] Alexandra L. Halberstadt[a]

[a]Department of Psychology, Pennsylvania State University, University Park, PA, USA; [b]Department of Clinical Psychology, Graduate School of Applied and Professional Psychology, Rutgers University, Piscataway, NJ, USA

Keywords

DSM-5 Alternative Model for Personality Disorders · Interpersonal behavior · Personality processes · Personality structure · Self and other

Abstract

Criteria A of the DSM-5 Alternative Model for Personality Disorders (AMPD) defines personality pathology in terms of impairments in "self" (identity, self-direction) and "interpersonal" (empathy, intimacy) functioning. Articulated as a set of dynamic regulatory and relational processes that are stratified in the Level of Personality Functioning Scale, these impairments involve how individuals think and feel about themselves and others and how they relate to others. Defining personality pathology in terms of regulatory and relational processes involving self and other, and distinguishing severity of personality pathology from individual differences in its expression (Criteria B), offers the AMPD several advantages. First, it distinguishes the nature and severity of personality pathology from other forms of psychopathology. Second, it allows the AMPD to integrate personality structure and personality processes. Third, it is highly suitable for synthesis with the Contemporary Integrative Interpersonal Theory of personality. Finally, beyond the interpersonal perspective, it facilitates even broader theoretical and treatment integration.

Introduction

In discussing the clinical science of personality disorders in the post-DSM-III/IV era, Pincus [1] distinguished defining what personality pathology is from describing individual differences in its expression, and further suggested that improvements in the classification of personality disorders "will require greater coordination of definitional theories and systems for describing variation in expression of personality pathology" (p. 287). This approach, which can also be conceived of as distinguishing the genus of personality pathology and the species of personality disorder [2, 3], is also reflected in the DSM-5 Alternative Model for Personality Disorders (AMPD) [4, 5]. Criteria A of the AMPD assesses what is common among all patients with personality pathology (genus) and Criteria B assesses individual differences in the expression of personality disorder (species).

Criteria A of the AMPD defines personality pathology in terms of impairments in "self" (identity, self-direction) and "interpersonal" (empathy, intimacy) functioning. Articulated as a set of dynamic regulatory and relational processes that are stratified in the Level of Personality Functioning Scale (LPFS) [4], these impairments involve how individuals think and feel about themselves and others and how they relate to others [6]. Although AMPD Criteria A semantics differentiates self and interpersonal

karger@karger.com
www.karger.com/psp

Karger

Aaron L. Pincus, PhD
Department of Psychology, Pennsylvania State University
358 Moore Bldg.
University Park, PA 16802 (USA)
aaron.l.pincus@gmail.com

impairments, self and other are intertwined throughout Criteria A diagnostic features (e.g., "Depends excessively on others for identity, self-esteem, and emotion regulation with compromised boundaries"; "Hyper-attuned to others, but only with respect to perceived relevance to self") and the LPFS renders a single rating of the severity of personality pathology. Conceptualizing the genus of personality pathology in terms of regulatory and relational processes involving self and other offers the AMPD several advantages. First, it distinguishes the nature and severity of personality pathology from other forms of psychopathology [7]. Second, it allows the AMPD to integrate personality structure and personality processes [8]. Third, it is highly suitable for synthesis with the Contemporary Integrative Interpersonal Theory (CIIT) of personality [9]. Finally, beyond the interpersonal perspective, it facilitates even broader theoretical and treatment integration [10, 11]. In the remainder of this paper, we discuss and elaborate these advantages.

Defining Personality Pathology and Its Severity

Self and interpersonal functioning deficits are the core feature of personality pathology, and it is the centrality of these impairments in self and other functioning that distinguishes personality pathology from other classes of psychopathology (e.g., eating, mood, anxiety, psychotic, substance use disorders, etc.) [7]. A growing number of empirical studies support this distinction. Scores on measures of psychosocial functioning significantly differ between those who do and those who do not have personality disorders [12–14], and scores on the LPFS itself reliably distinguish those who have a diagnosed personality disorder from those who do not [15]. In addition, using a bottom-up approach, factor analysis of diagnostic criteria for personality disorders yields a general personality disorder factor that maps well onto concepts in Criteria A [16]. Criteria A is often referred to as the "severity" indicator of the AMPD. Defining the severity of personality pathology in terms of impairments in self and other functioning common to all personality disorders, and distinguishing severity of personality pathology from individual differences in expression of personality disorder, are improvements over the DSM-5 Section II categorical diagnostic system for personality disorders where high severity is likely to lead to the undesirable outcome of meeting criteria for multiple personality disorder diagnoses [17].

This approach also has implications for patients' current and prospective functioning. Research supports the criterion validity and predictive validity of personality pathology severity [18]. Several studies demonstrate that general severity of personality pathology exhibits significant concurrent negative associations with psychosocial functioning in a broad range of domains, and many find that severity exhibits stronger and more pervasive associations with functional impairments than stylistic features of personality disorders [17, 19–22]. Importantly, longitudinal studies also support the predictive validity of general personality pathology severity over years [17, 19, 22] and the LPFS itself over days or weeks [23, 24]. Here we emphasize research that finds severity of personality pathology (including Criteria A LPFS) distinguishes personality disorders from other disorders and relates to current and prospective functioning regardless of, and sometimes more strongly than, stylistic features of personality disorders. Our discussion of severity does not address the contentious issue of overlap between Criteria A impairments and Criteria B traits [for reviews see 25, 26]. However, we believe the additional advantages of defining personality pathology and its severity with reference to self and other impairments discussed below further support DSM-5 AMPD Criteria A.

Integrating Personality Structure and Personality Processes

Integrating between-person personality trait structure and within-person dynamic personality processes can provide a more evidence-based and clinically useful model for conceptualizing and diagnosing personality disorders than using models based on structure or process alone [8, 27]. Personality traits are a fundamental component of personality disorders and are optimal for describing individual differences between patients. However, profiles of maladaptive trait elevations are not the clinical entities seen in the consulting room. Clinicians providing treatment primarily focus on regulatory and relational processes that unfold over time and serve as etiological and maintenance mechanisms for psychopathology. Individual differences in personality traits provide important information about the evoking contexts and style of expression of personality impairments, differentiating the species of personality disorder across patients. This added specificity can help focus and tailor psychotherapy given that most techniques of evidence-based treatments for personality disorders broadly target the impaired processes of the personality pathology genus, such as promoting accurate perceptions of self and other via mentalization in Transference-Focused Psychotherapy or im-

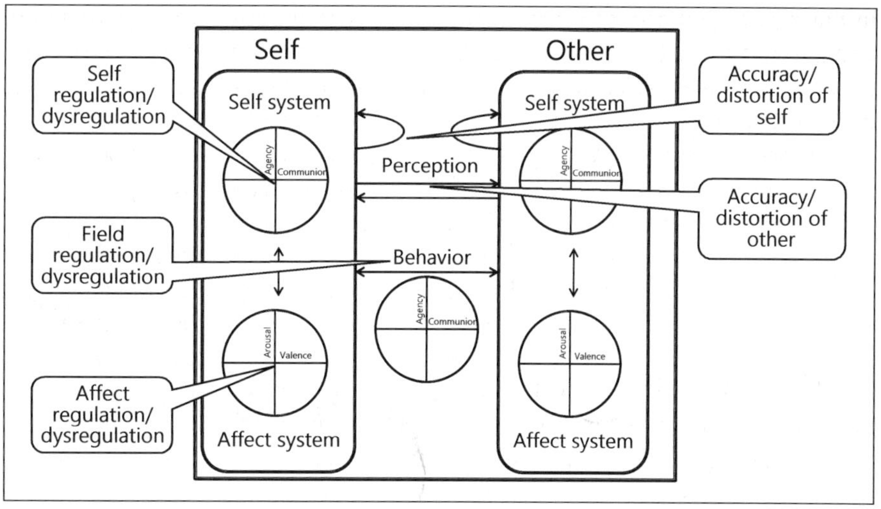

Fig. 1. The interpersonal situation.

proving emotion regulation via mindfulness in Dialectical Behavior Therapy. A patient's trait profile can help the clinician better predict how, and under what circumstances, the patient is likely to exhibit personality impairments [23], further informing intervention [11, 28]. A comprehensive approach that integrates assessment of individual differences with intensive repeated assessments of psychosocial functioning [e.g., 29–31] helps bring personality traits from bench to bedside [32, 33].

An Interpersonal Perspective on Criteria A

The AMPD attempts to integrate clinical theories of pathological personality processes (found in Criteria A) with an empirically derived dimensional trait model (found in Criteria B). However, this system is not well integrated into a cohesive framework sufficiently buttressed by clinical theory and research. Fortunately, the emphasis on self and other impairments in Criteria A allows for integration with existing theories of personality and paradigms of personality assessment with their rich empirical and clinical foundations [34]. One well-established theoretical framework that is highly compatible with an emphasis on self and other impairments is CIIT [9]. According to CIIT, agency and communion are the two core metaconstructs that underlie interpersonal experience. Together, agency and communion form a superordinate structure referred to as the Interpersonal Circumplex. This empirically derived structure is a focus of convenience that coordinates CIIT's dispositional (personality trait) and dynamic (personality process) features through the interpersonal situation framework [27, 35] (Fig. 1).

Interpersonal theory understands normal and disturbed interpersonal functioning in terms of the level and pervasiveness of distortion and dysregulation in interpersonal situations [1, 10]. Dysfunctional interpersonal styles reflect consistent patterns of regulatory and relational processes in interpersonal situations. Several potential foci are elaborated in Figure 1. Self-regulation involves the ability to effectively manage one's social cognition and self-concept, or how one thinks about oneself in relation to others in interpersonal situations. Affect regulation involves the ability to modulate one's inner emotional states and affective expression, or how one feels in interpersonal situations. Field regulation involves modulating the processes by which one relates to others in social transactions, or how one behaves and impacts others' behavior in interpersonal situations. Table 1 creates a crosswalk between AMPD Criteria A and the contemporary interpersonal model of personality pathology.

To bring this model to life, consider the individual with paranoid personality disorder and the recurrent interpersonal situation that characterizes their life (Fig. 2). Because the paranoid individual is high on the trait of suspiciousness, they are hypervigilant to threats from others and tend to distort perceptions of their behavior and motivation. For example, the coworker who genuinely offers collaboration is perceived as trying to steal ideas or unfairly take credit. This distorted view of the other as exploitative evokes dysregulated affect (anger), the motive to protect the self (remove the threat), and hostile interpersonal behavior that is consistent with the paranoid distortion and dysregulation but inconsistent with the genuine agentic and communal goals of the rebuffed coworker. In response, the coworker may respond

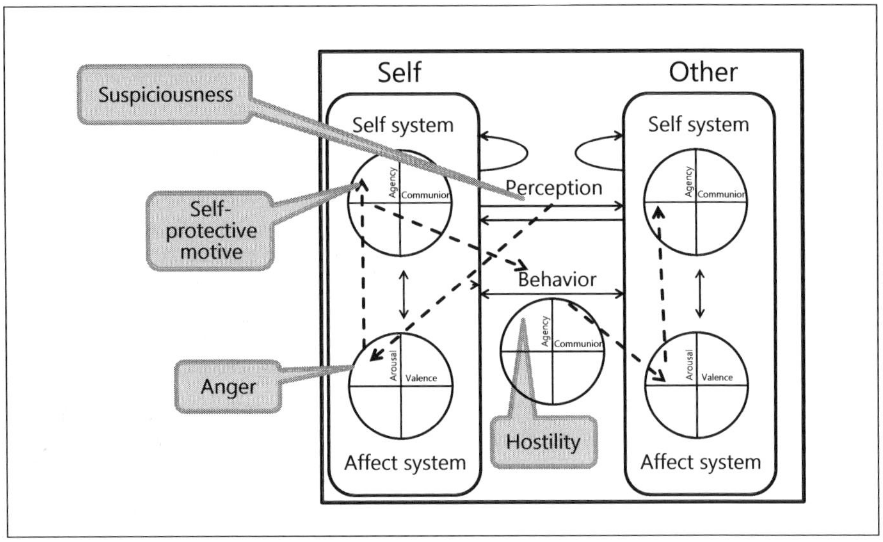

Fig. 2. The paranoid process.

Table 1. DSM-5 Alternative Model for Personality Disorders (AMPD) Criteria A crosswalk with interpersonal dysregulation and distortion

Interpersonal dysfunction	DSM-5 AMPD personality impairments
Distortion	*Identity:* Accuracy of self-appraisal and self-esteem *Self-Direction:* Ability to productively self-reflect *Empathy:* Comprehension of others' experiences *Empathy:* Understanding social causality *Empathy:* Comprehension of others' motivations
Self dysregulation	*Identity:* Experiences self as unique, with boundaries between self and others *Identity:* Coherent sense of time and personal history *Identity:* Stability of self-appraisal and self-esteem *Self-Direction:* Pursuit of coherent and meaningful short-term and life goals
Field dysregulation	*Self-Direction:* Uses constructive and prosocial internal standards of behavior *Empathy:* Understanding social causality *Empathy:* Tolerance of others' different perspectives *Intimacy:* Desire and capacity for closeness *Intimacy:* Deep and durable connections with others
Affect dysregulation	*Identity:* Capacity for a range of emotional experience and its regulation *Identity:* Capacity to regulate emotional experience and expression

with anger in kind or simply withdraw and not approach again. Regardless, a potentially creative collaboration was thwarted, and employee morale may be damaged. Distortion and dysregulation in interpersonal situations may be episodic and stress-induced (e.g., exhaustion and illness may create transient states of hypersensitivity) or chronic and pervasive (e.g., personality pathology).

The interpersonal situation coordinates empirically supported structures and processes from the CIIT perspective, and this can be expanded to the AMPD by similarly coordinating Criteria B (structure) and Criteria A (processes). Many of the Criteria A impairments in self and interpersonal functioning conceptually align themselves with agency and communion, respectively [2, 36]. Importantly, research finds that in social interactions in daily life, overall severity of personality impairment [37], stylistic features of personality disorders such as narcissism [38], and AMPD Criteria B traits such as antagonism [39] all impact patients' perceptions of self and other as agentic and communal, affective experiences, and functioning [for a review see 40]. The interpersonal model of personality pathology appears well suited to the task of integrating structure and process in the AMPD.

Clinical Theory and Clinical Practice

Beyond links to CIIT, Criteria A's focus on self and other impairments has additional advantages for theoretical integration and therapeutic practice. As noted above, many theories and evidence-based treatments for personality disorders already broadly focus on targeting self and other impairments. In fact, the authors of Criteria A drew on psychodynamic, attachment, interpersonal, and social-cognitive perspectives to develop the LPFS [6]. This pantheoretical approach to understanding general personality pathology severity in Criteria A maximizes treatment options for personality pathology across different theoretical models. For example, Transference-Focused Psychotherapy (TFP) [41] specifically targets the self-other dysfunction assessed by Criteria A by understanding and articulating the patient's mental representations of self, their mental representations of others, and the dominant affects that link these mental representations (e.g., a scared, victimized self representation linked to a sadistic, abusive other representation via fear). Through a series of clarifications, confrontations, and interpretations, the TFP therapist uses the here-and-now therapeutic relationship to increase the patient's awareness of and capacity to reflect on their self and interpersonal difficulties.

In Mentalization-Based Treatment (MBT) [42], the focus centers on increasing the patient's capacity for mentalization, or the ability to attend to and understand the mental states of self and other. MBT therapists actively focus on the patient's current mental state (their thoughts, feelings, wishes, desires) with the aim of building more adaptive internal states as well as better understanding of other's internal states. Disruptions in mentalization within the therapeutic relationship (i.e., shifts to non-mentalizing modes of experience) are inevitable and serve as key opportunities to work collaboratively to understand the interpersonal situation and affects immediately preceding the disruption.

Cognitive behavioral treatments for personality disorder also focus on the centrality of self-other difficulties found in Criteria A. For example, Schema-Focused Therapy (SFT) [43] argues that personality disorder arises from early maladaptive schemas about self and other that lead to rigid and enduring patterns of avoidance. An SFT therapist would use intervention techniques from behavioral, psychodynamic, and interpersonal treatment models to decrease the patient's avoidance and develop more adaptive schemas of self and other. Dialectical Behavior Therapy (DBT) [44] uses the biosocial theory to describe how the combination of biological (temperamental) vulnerability and an invalidating social environment leads to emotion regulation difficulties. DBT includes treatment strategies that emphasize more adaptive self and interpersonal functioning, such as mindfulness, validation, acceptance, distress tolerance, emotion regulation skills, and interpersonal skills. The DBT therapist aims to articulate unverbalized emotions, thoughts, or behavior patterns about self and other and communicates how current impairments in self and interpersonal functioning make sense given past social learning in the invalidating environment.

Having noted that multiple theories and treatment models specifically address self and other impairments, we also wish to highlight how the pantheoretical approach of the AMPD is consistent with the tenets of psychotherapy integration. Clarkin and colleagues [45] describe an integrated modular approach to the treatment of personality pathology that emphasizes (a) the individuality of the patient, not the category of the disorder; (b) the severity of dysfunction (Criteria A) and the specific expressions of dysfunction (Criteria B); (c) the therapeutic use of modules of intervention from existing evidence-based clinical approaches; and (d) intervention in the context of a developing alliance between therapist and patient. In this way, clinicians can integrate different evidence-based treatment techniques to address general personality severity and specific expressions of dysfunction. For example, a therapist might use the skills of DBT to help their patient to better understand and change their emotions while also using interventions from MBT to increase the patient's awareness of and mentalization about how their maladaptive views of self and other are contributing to their emotion dysregulation. As clinicians from diverse theoretical backgrounds begin to use the AMPD for treatment planning, research should focus on the genus (Criteria A) of personality pathology and the species of personality disorder (Criteria B) and how an integrated treatment approach can be used to target both severity of impairments and the specific expressions of dysfunction.

Conclusions

The clinical science undergirding classification, diagnosis, and treatment of personality disorders has become increasingly energized and diversified since the recognition of serious limitations of the DSM categorical nosology. By defining personality pathology in terms of self and other impairments and distinguishing severity of personality pathology from individual differences in its expression, the DSM-5 AMPD is a significant, if imperfect, step forward. The centrality of self and other impairments in Criteria A provides a focus that (a) distinguishes the core features of personality pathology from peripheral psychopathological symptoms that commonly co-occur with personality pathology (e.g., depressed mood, binge eating), (b) allows for an organic pantheoretical integration of perspectives on normal and abnormal personality, and (c) aligns with the intervention targets of evidence-based treatments for personality disorders and those of practicing clinicians more generally. Finally, when combined with the Criteria B traits, the Criteria A self and other impairments can be functionally linked within emerging frameworks integrating personality structure and personality processes [10, 46–48].

Additional work is needed to take full advantage of the AMPD's potential. First, we note that one area that has been extensively investigated is the cross-sectional overlap and incremental validity of Criteria A and Criteria B [25, 26]. Our view is that battles for cross-sectional incremental validity of traits and personality functioning measures have their place but generate negligible clinical insights. Why would we expect or require personality dysfunction and individual differences in personality to be orthogonal? Extraversion and neuroticism are known to be aspects of well-being for nearly 40 years [49], yet there are not calls to reduce the concept of well-being to profiles of trait elevations. We see such links as necessary not problematic, as personality traits and personality processes are not orthogonal. Thus, we agree with Hopwood's assertion that "further work focused on validating cross-sectional PD assessments and/or debating which traits underlie different PDs will not move the field forward" [32, p. 499]. Fortunately, the AMPD provides an ideal focus for clinical personality science to move forward by employing new longitudinal methodologies and dynamic statistical analyses that can truly model personality structure and personality processes [31, 37, 50–53]. Such work should also inform and be informed by clinical practice as efforts to develop more effective interventions for personality pathology continue. Future therapy approaches that target core self and other impairments and maladaptive traits, as well as tailor interventions with reference to severity of personality pathology and the patient's trait profile would serve to advance the next generation of treatment models [54–56]. These and related future advancements are facilitated by defining personality pathology in terms of personality processes reflecting impairments in self and other functioning and distinguishing the severity of personality impairment from individual differences in its expression [1].

Acknowledgements

We are grateful to our colleagues Dr. Christopher Hopwood and Dr. Aidan Wright for their continuing scholarly contributions to Contemporary Integrative Interpersonal Theory and the interpersonal situation framework.

Disclosure Statement

The authors have no conflicts of interest to declare.

Author Contributions

Each author contributed original drafts of specific sections of the manuscript.

References

1 Pincus AL. A Contemporary Integrative Interpersonal Theory of Personality Disorders. In: Lenzenweger MF, Clarkin JF, editors. Major Theories of Personality Disorder. 2nd ed. New York: Guilford Press; 2005. pp. 282–331.
2 Pincus AL. Some comments on nomology, diagnostic process, and narcissistic personality disorder in the DSM-5 proposal for personality and personality disorders. Pers Disord. 2011 Jan;2(1):41–53.
3 Pincus AL. In through the out door: a commentary on "personality disorders are the vanguard of the post-DSM-5.0 era". Pers Disord. 2013 Oct;4(4):363–4.
4 American Psychiatric Association. Diagnostic and Statistical Manual of Mental Disorders. 5th ed. Arlington (VA): American Psychiatric Association; 2013.
5 Skodol AE. Personality disorders in DSM-5. Annu Rev Clin Psychol. 2012;8(1):317–44.
6 Bender DS, Morey LC, Skodol AE. Toward a model for assessing level of personality functioning in DSM-5, part I: a review of theory and methods. J Pers Assess. 2011 Jul;93(4):332–46.
7 Hopwood CJ, Wright AG, Ansell EB, Pincus AL. The interpersonal core of personality pathology. J Pers Disord. 2013 Jun;27(3):270–95.
8 Hopwood CJ, Zimmermann J, Pincus AL, Krueger RF. Connecting personality structure and dynamics: towards a more evidence-based and clinically useful diagnostic scheme. J Pers Disord. 2015 Aug;29(4):431–48.
9 Dawood S, Dowgwillo EA, Wu LZ, Pincus AL. Contemporary integrative interpersonal theory of personality. In: Ziegler-Hill V, Shackelford, TK, editors. The SAGE Handbook of Personality and Individual Differences: Volume I: The Science of Personality and Individual Differences. London: SAGE Publications Ltd; 2018. p. 171–202. https://doi.org/10.4135/9781526451163.n8.

10 Pincus AL, Hopwood CJ. A contemporary interpersonal model of personality pathology and personality disorder. In: Widiger TA, editor. Oxford Handbook of Personality Disorders. New York (NY): Oxford University Press; 2012. pp. 372–98.
11 Hopwood CJ. A framework for treating DSM-5 alternative model for personality disorder features. Pers Ment Health. 2018 May;12(2):107–25.
12 DeFife JA, Goldberg M, Westen D. Dimensional assessment of self- and interpersonal functioning in adolescents: implications for DSM-5's general definition of personality disorder. J Pers Disord. 2015 Apr;29(2):248–60.
13 Beeney JE, Lazarus SA, Hallquist MN, Stepp SD, Wright AG, Scott LN, et al. Detecting the presence of a personality disorder using interpersonal and self-dysfunction. J Pers Disord. 2019 Apr;33(2):229–48.
14 Kampe L, Zimmermann J, Bender D, Caligor E, Borowski AL, Ehrenthal JC, et al. Comparison of the Structured DSM-5 Clinical Interview for the Level of Personality Functioning Scale with the Structured Interview of Personality Organization. J Pers Assess. 2018 Nov-Dec;100(6):642–9.
15 Morey LC, Bender DS, Skodol AE. Validating the proposed diagnostic and statistical manual of mental disorders, 5th edition, severity indicator for personality disorder. J Nerv Ment Dis. 2013 Sep;201(9):729–35.
16 Sharp C, Wright AG, Fowler JC, Frueh BC, Allen JG, Oldham J, et al. The structure of personality pathology: both general ('g') and specific ('s') factors? J Abnorm Psychol. 2015 May;124(2):387–98.
17 Hopwood CJ, Malone JC, Ansell EB, Sanislow CA, Grilo CM, McGlashan TH, et al. Personality assessment in DSM-5: empirical support for rating severity, style, and traits. J Pers Disord. 2011 Jun;25(3):305–20.
18 Skodol AE. Impact of personality pathology on psychosocial functioning. Curr Opin Psychol. 2018 Jun;21:33–8.
19 Wright AG, Hopwood CJ, Skodol AE, Morey LC. Longitudinal validation of general and specific structural features of personality pathology. J Abnorm Psychol. 2016 Nov;125(8):1120–34.
20 Buer Christensen T, Eikenaes I, Hummelen B, Pedersen G, Nysæter TE, Bender DS, et al. Level of personality functioning as a predictor of psychosocial functioning – Concurrent validity of criterion A [internet]. Pers Disord. 2019 Oct 3 [cited 2019 Nov 15] https://doi.org/10.1037/per0000352; advance online publication.
21 Roche MJ, Jacobson NC, Phillips JJ. Expanding the validity of the Level of Personality Functioning Scale observer report and self-report versions across psychodynamic and interpersonal paradigms. J Pers Assess. 2018 Nov-Dec;100(6):571–80.
22 Woods WC, Wright AG, Skodol AE, Morey LC, Hopwood CJ. Deconstructing individual differences in long-term personality disorder and trait change. Clin Psychol Sci. 2020 Jan;8(1):184–97.
23 Roche MJ, Jacobson NC, Pincus AL. Using repeated daily assessments to uncover oscillating patterns and temporally-dynamic triggers in structures of psychopathology: applications to the DSM-5 alternative model of personality disorders. J Abnorm Psychol. 2016 Nov;125(8):1090–102.
24 Roche MJ. Examining the alternative model for personality disorder in daily life: evidence for incremental validity. Pers Disord. 2018 Nov;9(6):574–83.
25 Zimmermann J, Kerber A, Rek K, Hopwood CJ, Krueger RF. A brief but comprehensive review of research on the Alternative DSM-5 Model for Personality Disorders. Curr Psychiatry Rep. 2019 Aug;21(9):92.
26 Widiger TA, McCabe GA. The AMPD from the perspective of the Five-factor Model. Psychopathology. Forthcoming 2020.
27 Hopwood CJ, Pincus AL, Wright AG. The interpersonal situation: integrating personality assessment, case formulation, and intervention. In: Samuel DB, Lynam DR, editors. Using basic Personality Research to Inform Personality Pathology [Internet] New York (NY): Oxford University Press; 2019 Feb. pp. 94–121. [cited 2019 Nov 15], available from https://www.oxfordclinicalpsych.com/view/10.1093/med-psych/9780190227074.001.0001/med-9780190227074-chapter-5.
28 Pincus AL, Dowgwillo EA, Greenberg LS. Three cases of narcissistic personality disorder through the lens of the DSM-5 Alternative Model for Personality Disorders. Pract Innov (Wash D C). 2016 Sep;1(3):164–77.
29 Roche MJ, Pincus AL. Precision assessment: An individualized and temporally dynamic approach to understanding patients in their daily lives. In: Kumar U, editor. The Wiley Handbook of Personality Assessment. Hoboken (NJ): Wiley Blackwell; 2016. pp. 192–204.
30 Wright AG, Zimmermann J. Applied ambulatory assessment: integrating idiographic and nomothetic principles of measurement. Psychol Assess. 2019 Dec;31(12):1467–80.
31 Zimmermann J, Woods WC, Ritter S, Happel M, Masuhr O, Jaeger U, et al. Integrating structure and dynamics in personality assessment: first steps toward the development and validation of a personality dynamics diary. Psychol Assess. 2019 Apr;31(4):516–31.
32 Hopwood CJ. Interpersonal dynamics in personality and personality disorders. Eur J Pers. 2018 Sep;32(5):499–524.
33 Pincus AL. Bringing personality traits from bench to bedside. Eur J Pers. 2018 Sep;32(5):572–3.
34 Pincus AL, Roche MJ. Paradigms of personality assessment and level of personality functioning (Criterion A) in the DSM-5 Alternative Model for Personality Disorders. In: Hopwood CJ, Mulay AL, Waugh MH, editors. The DSM-5 Alternative Model for Personality Disorders: Integrating Multiple Paradigms of Personality Assessment. New York: Routledge; 2019. pp. 48–59.
35 Pincus AL, Hopwood CJ, Wright AG. The interpersonal situation: an integrative framework for the study of personality, psychopathology, and psychotherapy. In: Rauthmann JF, Sherman RA, Funder DC, editors. The Oxford Handbook of Psychological Situations [Internet] New York (NY): Oxford University Press; 2017 Jun [cited 2019 Nov 15], available from https://www.oxfordhandbooks.com/view/10.1093/oxfordhb/9780190263348.001.0001/oxfordhb-9780190263348-e-4.
36 Dowgwillo EA, Roche MJ, Pincus AL. Examining the interpersonal nature of Criterion A of the DSM–5 Section III Alternative Model for Personality Disorders using bootstrapped confidence intervals for the interpersonal circumplex. J Pers Assess. 2018 Nov-Dec;100(6):581–92.
37 Dowgwillo EA, Pincus AL, Newman MG, Wilson SJ, Molenaar PC, Levy KN. Two methods for operationalizing the interpersonal situation to investigate personality pathology and interpersonal perception in daily life. In: Truslow LI, Rahmaan JM, editors. Personality disorders: What we know and future directions for research. New York: Nova Science Publishers; 2019. pp. 31–106.
38 Wright AG, Stepp SD, Scott LN, Hallquist MN, Beeney JE, Lazarus SA, et al. The effect of pathological narcissism on interpersonal and affective processes in social interactions. J Abnorm Psychol. 2017 Oct;126(7):898–910.
39 Wright AG. Antagonism from the perspective of interpersonal theory. In: Miller JD, Lynam DR, editors. The Handbook of Antagonism: Conceptualization, Assessment, Consequences, and Treatment at the Low End of Agreeableness. New York (NY): Academic Press; 2019. pp. 155–70.
40 Pincus AL. An interpersonal perspective on Criterion A of the DSM-5 Alternative Model for Personality Disorders. Curr Opin Psychol. 2018 Jun;21:11–7.
41 Caligor E, Kernberg OF, Clarkin JF, Yeomans FE. Psychodynamic psychotherapy for personality pathology: Treating self and interpersonal functioning. Washington (DC): American Psychiatric Association Publishing; 2018.
42 Bateman A, Fonagy P. Mentalization-based treatment for personality disorders: A practical guide. Oxford University Press; 2016. https://doi.org/10.1093/med:psych/9780199680375.001.0001.
43 Young JE, Klosko JS, Weishaar ME. Schema therapy: A practitioner's guide. New York (NY): The Guilford Press; 2003.
44 Lynch TR, Trost WT, Salsman N, Linehan MM. Dialectical behavior therapy for borderline personality disorder. Annu Rev Clin Psychol. 2007;3(1):181–205.
45 Clarkin JF, Cain N, Livesley WJ. An integrated approach to treatment of patients with personality disorders. J Psychother Integration. 2015 Mar;25(1):3–12.

46 Cervone D, Little BR. Personality architecture and dynamics: the new agenda and what's new about it. Pers Individ Dif. 2019 Jan;136: 12–23.
47 Jayawickreme E, Zachry CE, Fleeson W. Whole trait theory: an integrative approach to examining personality structure and process. Pers Individ Dif. 2019 Jan;136:2–11.
48 Huprich SK, Nelson SM. The cognitive-affective processing system model of personality pathology: Ready-made for theoretical integration. In: Huprich SK, editor. Personality disorders: Toward theoretical and empirical integration in diagnosis and assessment. Washington (DC): American Psychological Association; 2015. pp. 395–412.
49 Costa PT Jr, McCrae RR. Influence of extraversion and neuroticism on subjective well-being: happy and unhappy people. J Pers Soc Psychol. 1980 Apr;38(4):668–78.
50 Krueger RF. Personality disorders are the vanguard of the post-DSM-5.0 era. Pers Disord. 2013 Oct;4(4):355–62.
51 Ringwald WR, Hopwood CJ, Pilkonis PA, Wright AG. Dynamic features of affect and interpersonal behavior in relation to general and specific personality pathology. 2019. DOI: 10.31219/osf.io/4qevt.
52 Dotterer HL, Beltz AM, Foster KT, Simms LJ, Wright AG. Personalized models of personality disorders: using a temporal network method to understand symptomatology and daily functioning in a clinical sample. Psychol Med. 2019 Oct 10:1–9.
53 Sadler P, Woody E, McDonald K, Lizdek I, Little J. A lot can happen in a few minutes: examining dynamic patterns within an interaction to illuminate the interpersonal nature of personality disorders. J Pers Disord. 2015 Aug;29(4):526–46.
54 Clark LA, Nuzum H, Shapiro JL, Vanderbleek EN, Daly EJ, Simons AD, et al. Personality profiles as potential targets for intervention: identification and replication. Personal Ment Health. 2020 Feb;14(1):142–63.
55 Bach B, Bernstein DP. Schema therapy conceptualization of personality functioning and traits in ICD-11 and DSM-5. Curr Opin Psychiatry. 2019 Jan;32(1):38–49.
56 Rodriguez-Seijas, C, Ruggero, C, Eaton, NR, Krueger, RF. The DSM-5 Alternative Model for Personality Disorders and Clinical Treatment: A Review. Curr Treat Options Psych. 2019 Sept;6:284–98, https://doi.org/10.1007/s40501-019-00187-7.

Psychopathology

Review Article

Psychopathology 2020;53:141–148
DOI: 10.1159/000508353

Received: November 30, 2019
Accepted: April 16, 2020
Published online: July 22, 2020

An Object Relations Model Perspective on the Alternative Model for Personality Disorders (DSM-5)

John F. Clarkin[a] Eve Caligor[a, b] Julia F. Sowislo[a]

[a]Personality Disorders Institute and Department of Psychiatry, Weill Medical College of Cornell University, New York, NY, USA; [b]Department of Psychiatry, Vagelos College of Physicians and Surgeons of Columbia University, New York, NY, USA

Keywords

Alternative Model of DSM-5 · Object relations model · Personality disorders · Treatment of personality disorders

Abstract

The Alternative Model of DSM-5 combines dimensional ratings of self-functioning, interpersonal functioning, and traits with categorical classification. The object relations model has a long tradition pre-dating the Alternative Model and, in part, has been incorporated into the Alternative Model. The object relations model provides a theoretical background (generally missing in the Alternative Model) that enhances the clinical assessment of personality pathology and its relationship to treatment planning.

Introduction

The Alternative Model of DSM-5 Section III (AMPD) [1] with its hybrid approach to personality pathology is a work in progress, under theoretical scrutiny, subject to measurement development, and seeking acceptance by clinicians/researchers and the American Psychiatric Association. The hybrid approach combines six specific categories of personality disorder (antisocial, avoidant, borderline, narcissistic, obsessive-compulsive, and schizotypal personality disorder) defined by self- and interpersonal functioning with dimensional ratings and traits. This combination has been described as a clash of traditions in medicine and psychology [2]. It remains to be seen how the combination will enhance assessment and diagnosis of personality pathology.

In contrast, the object relations theory (ORT) model of personality pathology has an extensive history in clinical psychiatry [3] that foreshadowed and predated the AMPD. ORT involves the clinical recognition of observable categories (prototypes) of personality pathology (e.g., borderline and narcissistic personality disorder) while at the same time bringing attention to key domains of functioning that constitute personality pathology, and it can be assessed and measured dimensionally.

Our goal in this article is to compare the central aspects of the AMPD to those of ORT. We focus first on the AMPD with its general criteria for personality disorder and ratings of deficits in self-functioning and interpersonal functioning (criterion A) and pathological traits

karger@karger.com
www.karger.com/psp

Karger

John F. Clarkin
Westchester Division, New York Presbyterian Hospital
21 Bloomingdale Road
White Plains, NY 10605 (USA)
jclarkin@med.cornell.edu

(criterion B). We describe ORT, which has a long history in the psychoanalytic treatment tradition and combines attention to internal mental structure with related behavior. Finally, we compare the two models on key aspects of interest, including the definition of personality disorder, the ease and methods of assessment, and the model's relationship to treatment planning.

Description of and Rationale for the Alternative Model

The categorical diagnosis of personality disorders introduced in the DSM-III [4] and utilized in its subsequent versions was an impetus to empirical work on personality pathology but revealed a number of serious flaws in its application. These difficulties are well documented, including the heterogeneity within the individual diagnoses and the extensive co-morbidity among the disorders. Thus, the scene was set for major adjustments in the DSM-5, which resulted in conserving the categorical approach in the DSM-5 but including an Alternative Model in Section III, Emerging Measures and Models.

Dimensional Approach versus Categorical Approach

A primary intent of the DSM-5 initiative was to improve on the DSM-IV by an emphasis on dimensional measurement to more adequately capture the complexity and severity of pathology. The AMPD has taken the bold and controversial step of combining the categorical approach, describing six specific personality disorders, with dimensional measurement of self-functioning, interpersonal functioning, and traits. This has been called a clash of two traditions, the categorical tradition coming from medicine, and the dimensional, trait approach coming from academic psychology [2].

General Criteria for the Diagnosis of Personality Disorder

The AMPD has a number of criteria that capture the definition of personality disorder. Personality disorder involves the presence of significant impairments in self-functioning and interpersonal functioning. In addition, one or more pathological traits are present. The personality dysfunction described in this way is both inflexible and pervasive across a range of personal and social situations, and the dysfunction is relatively stable across time since adolescence or early adulthood.

Criterion A and Background Rationale. Criterion A defines the domains of self-functioning and interpersonal functioning that are seen as central to personality pathology. Self-functioning is specified as identity, self-direction (short- and long-term goals, standards of behavior, self-reflection), sense of self as a unique individual with clear boundaries, positive self-esteem, and accuracy of self-appraisal. Interpersonal functioning is defined by the capacity for empathy for and intimacy with others. A review of empirical data and theoretical writings showing the importance of self-functioning and interpersonal functioning to the overall severity of personality pathology was influential in the architecture of the AMPD [5]. This review noted that Kernberg's ORT was one of the first to articulate a model of personality types arrayed along a continuum of severity. This review led the way to the dimensional rating of self-functioning and interpersonal functioning, the Level of Personality Functioning Scale (LPFS).

Criterion B and Background Rationale. Criterion B is composed of five high-order traits: negative affect, detachment, antagonism, disinhibition, and psychoticism. These five higher-order traits have a number of related facets, not all of which are clearly indicated by the higher-order trait name. Negative affectivity, for example, includes facets of emotional lability, anxiousness, separation insecurity, submissiveness, hostility, and perseveration. The advantage of the multiple facets is coverage of numerous trait domains. A disadvantage is the lack of a theory that provides an indication of the overall importance of the multiple domains and facets to the functioning of the individual patient in his/her unique environment. Trait theory has a long tradition in clinical psychology for understanding and measuring personality functioning [6, 7]. A "trait" can be defined as a variable underlying a relatively stable disposition by the individual toward particular behavior patterns [7]. For example, the trait of aggression indicates that the individual is more likely than others who are lower on the trait dimension to exhibit behavior that is aggressive under stressful situations. The different traits are then used together to characterize an individual's functioning. There are a number of trait models, and the one adopted for the Alternative Model is conceptualized as a variant of the Big Five model. There are, however, a number of limitations in the trait approach in general, and in the use of a trait approach in the clinical assessment of patients [8]. Treatment is not focused on traits in the abstract, but rather on the triggers and contexts in which the disposition is turned into disruptive behavior. This requires that the clinical evaluation focus on the perceptions of the patient and the contexts in which the trait or disposition is activated.

Description of the ORT Model of Personality Pathology

The ORT model [9, 10] has its origins in the clinical understanding of patients engaged in intensive psychodynamic treatment and predates the theoretical focus on self-functioning and other functioning in the AMPD. The ORT of personality functioning and pathology is anchored in the construct of *identity*. Identity is the psychological structure seen to organize self- and interpersonal functioning, and pathology of identity formation seen as the defining feature of the personality disorders [3]. Normal identity formation, or *identity consolidation*, corresponds to a core sense of self that is stable, coherent, realistic, and continuous across time, a corresponding stable and rich experience of significant others, and an affective experience that is complex and well modulated. A coherent and integrated conception of self and others contributes to relationships that involve empathy and mutual dependence, as well as the ability to "mentalize," that is, to understand self and others in terms of intentions, motivations, and emotions.

In contrast, personality disorders at the level of borderline organization (e.g., borderline personality disorder) are characterized by pathology of identity formation, reflected in the absence of a fully elaborated, stable, and coherent core sense of self. In this setting, the experience of self and also of others is unstable, discontinuous, distorted, and poorly contextualized, and affects are poorly integrated and poorly modulated. Failure of identity consolidation is also associated with difficulty identifying and sustaining longer-term goals as well as with impaired capacity for empathy.

From a dynamic perspective, failure of identity formation reflects the impact of splitting-based or dissociative defenses, which interfere with normal integrative processes. Representations of self and others associated with positive affective experience are dissociated from those associated with negative affective experience. The resulting affectively charged, polarized internal representations fail to coalesce into an overarching sense of self and others. This is seen as accounting for the unstable and distorted sense of self and others that characterizes the personality disorders. In contrast, in normal identity formation, individual representations of self and others coalesce to form a coherent, integrated supraordinate sense of self, associated with both positive and negative affective experience and corresponding experience of significant others.

Classification of personality pathology within the framework of ORT focuses on core domains viewed as central to healthy personality functioning and disrupted in the personality disorders. Similar to the AMPD, the model emphasizes (1) identity formation (sense of self, sense of others, capacity to pursue longer-term personal goals) and (2) object relations (working models of relationships organizing interpersonal functioning). The ORT model is distinguished from the AMPD in that it also emphasizes the nature of (3) defensive operations, (4) the quality and management of aggression, (5) moral functioning and internalized values, and (6) reality testing as core determinants of personality functioning and the severity of personality pathology [9] (in the AMPD these features could be included as "trait specifiers"). Assessment of the nature and level of organization of functioning in these six domains provides both a dimensional profile of personality functioning and a determination of the individual's *personality organization*. Much as is seen in the LPFS, determination of personality organization, or the *level of personality organization*, can lead to classification of personality disorders on the basis of prototypes representing the severity of personality pathology falling across a continuous spectrum of pathology ranging from healthy personality functioning through severe pathology and linking its diagnostic classification to prognosis and treatment planning [10]. In the ORT model, severity of personality pathology is accompanied not only by deterioration of self- and interpersonal functioning as is noted in the AMPD, but also by deteriorating moral functioning (antisocial traits), increasing centrality of aggression (which may be self-directed as well as other-directed) in psychological functioning, and vulnerability of reality testing in the setting of extreme activation or conflict.

Because the ORT model has traditionally been focused on self (i.e., identity, defensive functioning, moral functioning, moderation of aggression) and functioning with others (i.e., quality of object relations) it has a close affinity with the AMPD. However, a major advantage of the ORT model is its theoretical and conceptual focus and clarity in contrast to the descriptive nature of the AMPD model. Clinical experience has confirmed that the five domains of functioning in ORT are central determinants of the level of organization and functioning of the individual with a close relationship to treatment focus and prognosis.

Comparison of the ORT Model with the AMPD

Aided by a background of information on both models of personality pathology and functioning, one can compare the two models on central aspects of interest.

Psychopathology 2020;53:141–148
DOI: 10.1159/000508353

Definition of Personality Disorder

A major contribution of the AMPD is a clear conception of the essence of personality pathology, which was missing in the DSM-III and its successors. The focus on self-functioning and functioning with others in interpersonal relations has theoretical and empirical support. The border between some difficulties and a personality disorder is clarified by the LPFS rating, which anchors the pathology with defined levels of severity.

The definition of personality disorder in ORT begins with a conceptualization of personality and normal personality functioning. Personality is the dynamic integration of behavior patterns derived from temperament, cognitive capacities, character and its subjective correlate of identity, and internalized value systems. A full view of personality must include the internal world of the individual and observable behavior patterns. Clinical assessment leads to a level of severity of difficulties in the organization of the personality, i.e., normal, neurotic, and high-, mid-, or low-level borderline organization. Consistent with the AMPD LPFS, moderate impairment is required for a personality disorder diagnosis. Thus, neurotic organization is considered subthreshold for the diagnosis, and a borderline level of organization at various levels of severity characterizes the personality disorders proper.

Domains of Functioning Relevant to the Two Models

There is, in fact, a considerable overlap between the domains of functioning as identified in AMPD criterion A and the domains of functioning privileged in the ORT model. Self-functioning in the AMPD is composed of identity and self-direction. These domains are captured extensively in the ORT model by Identity. The Interpersonal Functioning domain of the AMPD is composed of empathy and intimacy, both highlighted in the ORT domain of Object Relations. The five traits identified in the AMPD are evaluated in ORT by the domains of Aggression (negative affect), Object Relations (detachment, antagonism, disinhibition), and Reality Testing (psychoticism).

There are, however, several domains of functioning prominent in the ORT model that are not prominent in the alternative model. Defenses, spanning from normal defensive maneuvers and neurotic ones (rigidity, repression) to more extreme measures (e.g., splitting) are assessed in ORT. Furthermore, moral functioning, which can be variable in most personality disorders but is most evident in its absence in antisocial personality disorder, is an important domain of functioning in ORT. The ORT model posits that degrees of moral functioning deficits are involved not only in antisocial personality disorder but potentially also in all severe personality disorders, in particular among patients presenting with borderline, narcissistic, and paranoid personality disorders and malignant narcissism. In these disorders, the presence and extent of deficits in moral functioning serve as a robust marker of severity of personality pathology.

The two models arrived at their respective domains by different routes. The five domains of interest in the ORT model were derived from clinical experience and theoretical reflection on those domains of human functioning that are consistently related to personality pathology [3]. This theoretical formulation has been called upon to inform the selection of self-functioning and interpersonal functioning in AMPD criterion A.

In contrast, personality researchers emphasize that the higher-order traits included in AMPD criterion B are not based on mere theory but rather on a sound empirical approach. What is the foundation for this claim? The generation of traits is based upon a lexical examination of nouns and adjectives that describe human behavior. These items are placed in a self-report instrument and subjected to factor analysis to yield traits. This process is empirical in the sense that factor analysis is applied to the data. However, the data are typically self-report information from individuals, subject to the limitations of accuracy on the part of the respondent. Factor analysis is based on correlations between responses across the sample, and it not descriptive of any one individual.

Clinical Assessment

The time-honored assessment procedure between prospective patient and therapist is the clinical interview. The major goal of the clinical assessment is to provide a clear focus (to both the patient and the therapist) for the therapeutic intervention. Through the process of evaluation, patient and therapist come to a clearer and shared conceptualization of the targets of intervention and the patient's motivation for change. The clinical interview has the advantage of direct contact between patient and potential therapist and provides direct evidence of the quality of the patient's relations with others. An important practical issue is how the two different models would guide the clinical assessment interview.

There is little information on how the AMPD would guide the initial clinical interview in terms of organization and sequence. The content of the AMPD would dictate that the clinical interview pursues information concerning self-functioning (identity and self-direction) and important interactions with others in the individual's current environment (criterion A). There are several semi-structured interviews (detailed later in this article) that can guide the clinician in this process. This information would also inform the assessor's ratings of the traits in criterion B.

The structure and focus of the clinical assessment interview according to ORT is informed by the structural interview [3]. The sequence of this clinical but clearly defined interview proceeds from chief complaint and motivation for change, to prominent current symptoms, to the extent and quality of interpersonal relations. The yield of the interview is information that can be used to make a diagnosis of the type and severity of personality disorder. In cases of personality pathology where there are questions of possible thought disorder, deficits in cognitive functioning, etc., a more extensive assessment battery could be utilized.

Ancillary Assessment Procedures

Criterion A of the AMPD (i.e., severity) can be operationalized by ratings on the LPFS, either by an expert clinician, the participant her-/himself, or an informant [for an overview, see 11]. These ratings can be made either on a global level (i.e., single 5-point scale) or on a more differentiated level (i.e., separate ratings of the 4 domains, the 12 subdomains, or the 60 prototypical descriptions). Information relevant to the clinician ratings can be collected using one of several structured clinical interviews, such as the Structured Clinical Interview for the Level of Personality Functioning Scale [12] or the Semi-Structured Interview for Personality Functioning DSM-5 [13]. In addition to that, more recently, self-report measures corresponding to the LPFS have been developed. These include the Level of Personality Functioning Scale-Self Report [14] and its brief form [15], the DSM-5 Levels of Personality Functioning Questionnaire [16], and the Self and Interpersonal Functioning Scale [17].

Criterion B of the AMPD (i.e., maladaptive traits) can as well be operationalized by expert clinician report, self-report, or informant report. The most common way to measure criterion B is the Personality Inventory for DSM-5 [18], a 220-item self-report questionnaire which assesses the 25 facet traits and the 5 higher-order traits. Additionally, a short form with 100 items [19], a brief form with 25 items [20], and an informant report form [21] are available. Expert clinician ratings can be done using the Personality Trait Rating Form [22], which includes 25 items measuring the facet traits, whereby the necessary information for those ratings can be gained using the Structured Clinical Interview for Personality Traits [23]. These developing instruments for criteria A and B are useful for research, but their role in clinical practice will probably be minor, as most clinicians do not use questionnaires in routine practice and prefer the clinical interview.

The clinical assessment of patient symptoms and personality organization in ORT can be accomplished using the structural interview [3], and its semi-structured interview format as described in the Structured Interview for Personality Organization (STIPO) [24, 25] and the shorter revision, the STIPO-R [24]. The STIPO-R is not only useful for research, but it can also be a guide for the clinician performing an initial patient evaluation.

STIPO ratings of severity are consistent with diagnostic measures of pathology. The STIPO domains discriminate between clinical and nonclinical subjects. There is a significant correlation between personality organization on the STIPO and the number of SCID-II diagnoses. Patients with DSM personality disorder were found to be on a lower level of personality organization in all domains than were patients without personality disorder. Based on the domain ratings of the STIPO, a prototypical profile of borderline personality organization (BPO) was developed and tested in its ability to discriminate between BPO and non-BPO.

STIPO domain ratings are useful in assessing clinical engagement and change. For example, STIPO domains identify treatment dropout among dual-diagnosis patients more effectively than do personality disorder diagnoses. In a randomized clinical trial comparing transference-focused psychotherapy to treatment in the community by expert therapists, the STIPO detected change in personality organization in both groups, with superior change in the transference-focused psychotherapy group.

Description versus Hypothesized Connections

Traits (criterion B) are descriptions of action tendencies as reported by subjects on self-report questionnaires. Criterion A is a description of aspects of self- and interpersonal functioning. In contrast, ORT is a clinically based theoretical model that posits cause and effect between internalized object relations empowered by strong affects as they impact on the nature and quality of interactions between self and others. This type of model provides a road map for treatment intervention.

Table 1. Severity of personality pathology: implications for assessment and treatment parameters [10]

	Neurotic organization	High borderline personality organization	Mid borderline personality organization	Low borderline personality organization
Level of Personality Functioning Scale (LPFS)	Level 1	Level 2	Level 3	Level 4
Typical categorical diagnosis	Obsessive compulsive PD; depressive PD; hysterical PD	Dependent PD; histrionic PD; avoidant PD; narcissistic PD	Narcissistic PD; borderline PD; paranoid PD; schizoid PD	Narcissistic, borderline, and paranoid PDs with antisocial features; antisocial PD
Nature of self-other functioning	Integrated, realistic, and continuous experience of self in relation to others; relationships characterized by mutuality	Somewhat superficial and/or polarized experience of self in relation to others; some capacity for dependency but with conflict	Superficial, extreme, polarized, and unstable sense of self in relation to others with gross distortion; need-fulfilling relationships	Caricature-like, extreme, highly polarized, and chaotic sense of self in relation to others with gross distortion; exploitative relationships
Clinical objectives of treatment	Flexible functioning in area of conflict	Greater depth and stability in experience of self and others	Resolution of destructive behavior; greater depth in experience of self and others	Behavior control; modulation of aggression
Prognosis	Excellent	Good	Fair	Very guarded
Structuring of the treatment	Less need for structured contract	Explicitly agreed-upon treatment contract promotes productive clinical process	Carefully constructed treatment contract is essential	Contracting must be extensive; focus on secondary gain and safety of patient and therapist
Treatment process	Little to no risk of acting out	Risk of low-level acting out (e.g., poor attendance)	Risk of dangerous acting out (e.g., suicide gestures or attempts, substance misuse)	Potentially lethal acting out (e.g., threats of violence to therapist, lethal suicide attempts)
Alliance	Clarity about seeking help from expert; open to alliance	Ambivalence about seeking help and depending on expert interference with initial alliance; early alliance unstable or superficial	Suspicion, with fear of critical attack or exploitation by therapist interferes with alliance; alliance built during course of treatment	Relatively fixed view of therapist as corrupt, arrogant, and exploitative limits capacity to form an alliance

PD, personality disorder.

Contribution of the Assessment Process to Treatment Planning

An essential approach to the evaluation of a diagnostic system is to review its clinical utility: how well does it meet the needs of clinicians evaluating and treating patients. Aspects of clinical utility include user acceptability and utility, professional communication, interrater reliability, subtlety of diagnosis, and clinical decision-making [26]. The evidence for the clinical utility of the AMPD is just beginning to be accumulated, with evidence that clinicians prefer the emphasis on dimensional assessment [27].

A major consideration is the relevance of the assessment process to the clinician's articulation of a treatment plan, and the communication between clinician and patient concerning the need, focus, and process of treatment intervention. The relationship between the AMPD and treatment planning is only implicit and not articulated in the diagnostic manual. This gap in the diagnostic manual is understandable and fitting, as it is not the role of the AMPD to make choices between competing treatment orientations that must be judged empirically aside from the diagnostic process.

A major advantage of the ORT model is the direct linkages it makes between a theoretical focus on key domains of functioning, assessment techniques and methods, and treatment planning [24]. Table 1 describes the relationship between levels of personality organization, as revealed in the structural interview or in a clinical interview guided by the STIPO-R, and key aspects of the treatment process. The severity of the level of personality organization disturbance is directly related to the structure and focus of the therapeutic intervention.

Conclusions

The inclusion of the AMPD in the DSM-5 has provided a positive stimulus to refining our conceptions of personality pathology and its assessment. A primary concern in the evaluation of the AMPD is its suitability to be included as the official diagnostic system. Does it meet the clinical and administrative requirements for a diagnostic system [26]? At this point, it is our view that its central focus on self-functioning and functioning with others is a positive advance over the current system. In addition, the emphasis on dimensional ratings of domains of functioning (i.e., severity) is essential for treatment planning.

An important perspective, however, is an evaluation of the AMPD as an expression of how the field is advancing in the understanding of personality pathology. The debates over the AMPD go far beyond its value in diagnosing patients (the reporting of the diagnosis to insurance companies in the USA is done with the ICD-10) and attracts intense debate on the very nature and classification of personality pathology. It is this articulation of the growing view of personality pathology that is so important for the field. With the infusion of developing research, it is possible that the differences between two traditions in the AMPD can be transformed into a more integrated view.

Conflict of Interest Statement

The authors have no conflicts of interest to declare.

Funding Sources

This work was supported by a research grant from the Swiss National Science Foundation to J.F.S.

Author Contributions

J.F.C. drafted the manuscript. E.C. and J.F.S. critically revised the manuscript. All authors reviewed the final manuscript.

References

1 American Psychiatric Association. Diagnostic and statistical manual of mental disorders. 5th ed. Arlington (VA): American Psychiatric Association; 2013.

2 Kendler KS. Classification of psychopathology: conceptual and historical background. World Psychiatry. 2018 Oct;17(3):241–2.

3 Kernberg OF. Severe personality disorders: psychotherapeutic strategies. New Haven (CT): Yale University Press; 1984.

4 American Psychiatric Association. Diagnostic and statistical manual of mental disorders. 3rd ed. Arlington (VA): American Psychiatric Association; 1980.

5 Bender DS, Morey LC, Skodol AE. Toward a model for assessing level of personality functioning in DSM-5, part I: a review of theory and methods. J Pers Assess. 2011 Jul;93(4):332–46.

6 Kotov R, Krueger RF, Watson D, Achenbach TM, Althoff RR, Bagby RM, et al. The Hierarchical Taxonomy of Psychopathology (HiTOP): a dimensional alternative to traditional nosologies. J Abnorm Psychol. 2017 May;126(4):454–77.

7 Markon KE, Jonas KG. The role of traits in describing, assessing, and understanding personality pathology. In: Huprich SK, editor. Personality disorders: toward theoretical and empirical integration in diagnosis and assessment. Washington (D.C): American Psychological Association; 2015. pp. 63–84.

8 Meehan KB, Clarkin JF. A critical evaluation of moving toward a trait system for personality disorder assessment. In: Huprich SK, editor. Personality disorders: toward theoretical and empirical integration in diagnosis and assessment. Washington (D.C): American Psychological Association; 2015. pp. 85–106.

9 Kernberg OF, Caligor E. A psychodynamic theory of personality disorders. In: Lenzenweger MF, Clarkin JF, editors. Major theories of personality disorder. 2nd ed. New York (NY): Guilford Press; 2005. pp. 114–56.

10 Caligor E, Kernberg OF, Clarkin JF, Yeomans FE. Psychodynamic therapy for personality pathology: treating self and interpersonal functioning. Washington (D.C.): American Psychiatric Association Publishing; 2018.

11 Zimmermann J, Kerber A, Rek K, Hopwood CJ, Krueger RF. A brief but comprehensive review of research on the Alternative DSM-5 Model for Personality Disorders. Curr Psychiatry Rep. 2019 Aug;21(9):92.

12 Bender DS, Skodol AE, First MB, Oldham JM. Module I: Structured Clinical Interview for the Level of Personality Functioning Scale. In: First MB, Skodol AE, Bender DS, Oldham JM, editors. Structured Clinical Interview for the DSM-5 Alternative Model for Personality Disorders (SCID-AMPD). Arlington (VA): American Psychiatric Association Publishing; 2018.

13 Hutsebaut J, Kamphuis JH, Feenstra DJ, Weekers LC, De Saeger H. Assessing DSM-5-oriented level of personality functioning: development and psychometric evaluation of the Semi-Structured Interview for Personality Functioning DSM-5 (STiP-5.1). Personal Disord. 2017 Jan;8(1):94–101.

14 Morey LC. Development and initial evaluation of a self-report form of the DSM-5 Level of Personality Functioning Scale. Psychol Assess. 2017 Oct;29(10):1302–8.

15 Hutsebaut J, Feenstra DJ, Kamphuis JH. Development and preliminary psychometric evaluation of a brief self-report questionnaire for the assessment of the DSM-5 Level of Personality Functioning Scale: the LPFS Brief Form (LPFS-BF). Personal Disord. 2016 Apr; 7(2):192–7.

16 Huprich SK, Nelson SM, Meehan KB, Siefert CJ, Haggerty G, Sexton J, et al. Introduction of the DSM-5 Levels of Personality Functioning Questionnaire. Personal Disord. 2018 Nov;9(6):553–63.

17 Gamache D, Savard C, Leclerc P, Côté A. Introducing a short self-report for the assessment of DSM-5 level of personality functioning for personality disorders: the Self and Interpersonal Functioning Scale. Personal Disord. 2019 Sep;10(5):438–47.

18 Krueger RF, Derringer J, Markon KE, Watson D, Skodol AE. Initial construction of a maladaptive personality trait model and inventory for DSM-5. Psychol Med. 2012 Sep;42(9):1879–90.
19 Thimm JC, Jordan S, Bach B. The Personality Inventory for DSM-5 Short Form (PID-5-SF): psychometric properties and association with Big Five traits and pathological beliefs in a Norwegian population. BMC Psychol. 2016 Dec;4(1):61.
20 Bach B, Maples-Keller JL, Bo S, Simonsen E. The alternative DSM-5 personality disorder traits criterion: a comparative examination of three self-report forms in a Danish population. Personal Disord. 2016 Apr;7(2):124–35.
21 Markon KE, Quilty LC, Bagby RM, Krueger RF. The development and psychometric properties of an informant-report form of the Personality Inventory for DSM-5 (PID-5). Assessment. 2013 Jun;20(3):370–83.
22 Few LR, Miller JD, Rothbaum AO, Meller S, Maples J, Terry DP, et al. Examination of the Section III DSM-5 diagnostic system for personality disorders in an outpatient clinical sample. J Abnorm Psychol. 2013 Nov;122(4):1057–69.
23 Skodol AE, First MB, Bender DS, Oldham JM. Module II: Structured Clinical Interview for Personality Traits. In: First MB, Skodol AE, Bender DS, Oldham JM, editors. Structured Clinical Interview for the DSM-5 Alternative Model for Personality Disorders (SCID-AMPD). Arlington (VA): American Psychiatric Association Publishing; 2018.
24 Clarkin JF, Caligor E, Stern B, Kernberg OF. The Structured Interview of Personality Organization – Revised (STIPO-R). 2016. Available from: https://www.borderlinedisorders.com/structured-interview-of-personality-organization.php.
25 Hörz-Sagstetter S, Caligor E, Preti E, Stern BL, De Panfilis C, Clarkin JF. Clinician-guided assessment of personality using the Structural Interview and the Structured Interview of Personality Organization (STIPO). J Pers Assess. 2018 Jan–Feb;100(1):30–42.
26 Verheul R. Clinical utility of dimensional models for personality pathology. In: Widiger TA, Simonsen E, Sirovatka PJ, Regier DA, editors. Dimensional models of personality disorders: refining the research agenda for DSM-V. Washington (DC): American Psychiatric Association; 2006. pp. 203–18.
27 Bornstein RF, Natoli AP. Clinical utility of categorical and dimensional perspectives on personality pathology: a meta-analytic review. Personal Disord. 2019 Nov;10(6):479–90.

Psychopathology

Review Article

Psychopathology 2020;53:149–156
DOI: 10.1159/000507378

Received: December 2, 2019
Accepted: March 19, 2020
Published online: June 11, 2020

The Alternative Model of Personality Disorders (AMPD) from the Perspective of the Five-Factor Model

Thomas A. Widiger Gillian A. McCabe

Department of Psychology, University of Kentucky, Lexington, KY, USA

Keywords

DSM-5 · Alternative Model of Personality Disorders · AMPD · Five-Factor Model · Personality disorders · Personality traits

Abstract

The fifth edition of the American Psychiatric Association's (APA) *Diagnostic and Statistical Manual of Mental Disorders* (DSM-5; American Psychiatric Association. Diagnostic and Statistical Manual of Mental Disorders. 5th ed. Washington: American Psychiatric Association; 2013) includes an Alternative Model of Personality Disorders (AMPD). The AMPD includes two components: the Criterion A level of personality functioning (i.e., impairments or deficits in the sense of self and interpersonal relatedness) and the Criterion B five-domain maladaptive trait model. The purpose of the current paper is to discuss the AMPD from the perspective of the Five-Factor Model (FFM) of general personality structure. The conclusion of this review is that both the Criterion A self-other deficits and the Criterion B traits can be understood as maladaptive variants of the FFM.

The Alternative Model of Personality Disorders from the Perspective of the Five-Factor Model

The fifth edition of the American Psychiatric Association's (APA) *Diagnostic and Statistical Manual of Mental Disorders* (DSM-5; [1]) includes an Alternative Model of Personality Disorders (AMPD). The AMPD includes two components: (1) the Criterion A level of personality functioning (LPF; i.e., impairments or deficits in the sense of self and interpersonal relatedness) and (2) the Criterion B five-domain maladaptive trait model. The AMPD is a significant step toward the development of a dimensional trait model conceptualization of personality disorders (PDs) that will provide a more accurate, complete, and clinically useful description of a patient's personality, facilitating thereby patient-therapist communication and treatment planning [2–4]. The purpose of this paper is to discuss the AMPD from the perspective of the Five-Factor Model (FFM) of general personality structure. Both the Criterion A LPF and the Criterion B maladaptive trait model will be considered. We begin with a discussion of the relationship of the Criterion B traits with the FFM, as this relationship is relatively more straightforward.

karger@karger.com
www.karger.com/psp

Karger

Thomas A. Widiger, PhD
Department of Psychology
University of Kentucky, 115 Kastle Hall
Lexington, KY 40506-0044 (USA)
widiger@uky.edu

Criterion B: Maladaptive Personality Traits

The FFM is the predominant dimensional model of general personality structure [5, 6], consisting of the five broad domains of neuroticism (or emotional instability versus stability), extraversion (versus introversion), openness (or unconventionality), agreeableness (versus antagonism), and conscientiousness (or constraint versus disinhibition). The DSM-5 AMPD trait model includes the domains of negative affectivity, detachment, psychoticism, antagonism, and disinhibition [1]. As stated in the DSM-5, these "five broad domains are maladaptive variants of the five domains of the extensively validated and replicated personality model known as the "Big Five," or the Five Factor Model of personality" [1, p. 773].

It should be acknowledged though that when the trait model was first posted on the DSM-5 website in 2010 (consisting at that time of six domains), it was not aligned with the FFM. On the contrary, Clark and Krueger [7] explicitly distanced the DSM-5 trait model from the FFM, stating that compulsivity (which was included as a sixth domain) did not align with FFM conscientiousness and that schizotypy (which eventually became the psychoticism domain) did not align with FFM openness. For some, this gave the appearance that the model was created de nova (i.e., was not aligned with any existing trait model) and was not well grounded in the considerable body of prior FFM research [8, 9]. As expressed by Shedler et al. [10] in their *American Journal of Psychiatry* editorial objecting to the trait model, "the resulting model no longer rests on decades of research, which had been the chief rationale for including it" (p. 1027). However, in the end, the DSM-5 trait model was aligned with the FFM [1, p. 773]. As affirmed by Krueger and Markon [11], the DSM-5 trait "domains can be understood as maladaptive extremes of the five-factor model (FFM) that has usefully framed extensive research in the field of personality and individual differences" (p. 480).

The FFM traces its roots to the Big Five, a trait model derived from a factor analysis of virtually every trait term within the English and other languages [12]. To the extent that the Big Five includes every maladaptive trait term, it naturally follows that the FFM, aligned with the Big Five, accounts for virtually every maladaptive personality trait [6]. There is indeed a substantial body of research documenting that the FFM accounts for all of the DSM-IV PDs [2, 3]. Multiple persons who have reviewed the FFM-PD research have reached the conclusion that all of the PDs can be understood as maladaptive variants of the FFM (e.g., [4, 13–15]).

There are also now quite a few studies documenting the alignment of the DSM-5 trait model with the FFM (e.g., [16–26]). One point of dispute though has been the alignment of psychoticism with openness. Some studies have reported essentially no relationship (e.g., [24, 25, 27]); and even for many of the studies that have reported a relationship, the strength of the association has been relatively weak (e.g., [17, 19–21]). It is evident that the strength of the relationship of psychoticism with FFM openness depends substantially on how both openness and psychoticism are defined and/or assessed [28].

Openness

Costa and McCrae [29] began with just a three-factor model. Once they became aware of the Big Five, they expanded their model to include the domains of antagonism and conscientiousness, assessed by the NEO Personality Inventory-Revised (NEO PI-R; [30]). However, they did not revise their measure of neuroticism, extraversion, or openness to be optimally aligned with the respective Big Five domains of emotional instability, surgency, and intellect, respectively. This was not a problem for neuroticism and extraversion as they were already very closely congruent with the Big Five domains of emotional instability and surgency, but Costa and McCrae had conceptualized openness to emphasize ideal personality traits of self-actualization, an open mind, and self-realization, citing humanism papers and texts. This was not how the respective domain (i.e., intellect) was conceptualized within the Big Five. There was certainly a strong convergence of FFM openness with Big Five intellect, but there were also important differences. Big Five intellect is more heavily predominated by such traits as unconventionality, eccentricity, and nonconforming, along with an openness to values and feelings [31].

Alternative measures and models of openness have been developed for which a clearer relationship with schizotypal thinking has been more readily apparent, including the Odd and Eccentric scale developed by Piedmont and colleagues [32], Openness/Intellect within the Big Five Aspects scale [33], the Absorption scale within the 5-Dimensional Personality Test (5-DPT; [34]), the Unconventionality scale within the HEXACO-Personality Inventory (HEXACO-PI; [35]), and the Unconventionality domain within the Inventory of Personal Characteristics-5 (IPC-5; [36]). Tellegen [37] in fact suggested years ago with respect to his unconventionality conceptualization of openness that "markers of this type are clinically suggestive, particularly of schizotypal personality disorder" (p. 126).

The studies that have obtained the weakest relationship of openness with psychoticism have typically relied on a NEO inventory or a closely comparable measure (e.g., [22, 25, 27]). Positive results have been more consistently obtained with the alternative measures of openness (e.g., [19, 23, 38–42]). For example, Gore and Widiger [20] conducted a joint factor analysis of the Personality Inventory for DSM-5 (PID-5; [43]) that assessed the DSM-5 dimensional trait model, along with the IPC-5 of Tellegen and Waller [36] and the 5-DPT of van Kampen [34], as well as the NEO PI-R [30]. The optimal solution was a five-factor model, with an openness-psychoticism factor defined heavily by IPC-5 Unconventionality, 5-DPT Absorption, and PID-5 Psychoticism, as well as (but more weakly) by NEO PI-R Openness.

Psychoticism

The conceptualization and assessment of psychoticism is equally important [28]. The DSM-5 trait model organizes the maladaptive traits included within the DSM-IV PDs into the five trait domains [1]. DSM-5 AMPD antagonism, for example, includes traits from the narcissistic and antisocial PDs, as well as the paranoid, schizotypal, and (to a lesser extent) borderline. Psychoticism would be comparably defined largely by the cognitive, behavioral, and perceptual aberrations of the schizotypal PD (e.g., magical thinking and odd-eccentric behavior). The original name for this domain was indeed schizotypy [4]. However, the PID-5 assessment of psychoticism includes overt psychotic delusions. Schizotypal personality traits (e.g., eccentricity and magical ideation) are on a continuum with psychotic delusions, but there are important differences between a personality trait and a delusion. A fundamental and defining feature of a personality trait (and a PD) is an early onset and a largely chronic presence thereafter, whereas a delusion can appear at any point in a person's life and will be limited in its duration. Delusions are not typically understood to be personality traits and are not included within the diagnostic criteria for schizotypal PD [1]. Delusions are part of acute psychotic episodes.

Nevertheless, the PID-5 includes delusions within two of the three subscales (i.e., Cognitive and Perceptual Dysregulation and Unusual Beliefs and Experiences; PID-5 Eccentricity does not include any references to delusions). Three sample items are "Sometimes I feel 'controlled' by thoughts that belong to someone else," "Sometimes I think someone else is removing thoughts from my head," and "Sometimes I can influence other people just by sending my thoughts to them." And, these are not just mild delusions, these are Schneiderian delusions of thought control and thought broadcasting [44], considered at one time to be pathognomonic for schizophrenia and still considered today to represent the most severe forms of delusions [1, 44], well beyond the pathology evident within a schizotypal PD.

Crego and Widiger [40] administered the three PID-5 Psychoticism scales along with the three corresponding scales from the Five Factor Schizotypal Inventory (FFSI [45]; i.e., FFSI Aberrant Ideas, Aberrant Perceptions, and Odd and Eccentric). None of the FFSI scales includes references to delusions or hallucinations. Also included were two personality trait scales: IPIP-NEO Imagination [46] and IPC-5 Unconventionality [36] that assess for Big Five openness. All three of the FFSI schizotypal cognition-perception scales obtained medium to large effect size relationships with the personality traits of imagination and unconventionality, whereas PID-5 Cognitive and Perceptual Dysregulation and PID-5 Unusual Beliefs and Experiences were largely uncorrelated with the FFM traits. PID-5 Eccentricity, which does not include any references to psychotic delusions, did obtain medium to large effect size relationships with the FFM traits. In a joint factor analysis, the three FFSI schizotypal cognition-perception scales, PID-5 Eccentricity, IPIP-NEO Imagination, and IPC-5 Unconventionality defined a distinct openness-schizotypal factor, whereas PID-5 Cognitive and Perceptual Dysregulation and PID-5 Unusual Beliefs and Experiences, including the psychotic items, separated to form their own distinct factor. These results were closely replicated in a separate data collection, this time including HEXACO PI-R Unconventionality (instead of IPC-5 Unconventionality), along with the three FFSI schizotypal cognition-perception scales, the three PID-5 psychoticism scales, and IPIP-NEO Imagination [40].

Conclusions

In sum, the DSM-5 AMPD trait model can be understood as an instantiation of FFM PD [8]. There are, of course, other possible maladaptive trait models derived from the FFM. The FFM includes all possible maladaptive personality traits, with clearly many, many more traits than are included just within the DSM-5 Criterion B AMPD. Coker et al. [31] identified 803 maladaptive trait terms within the English language, and further indicated that there are maladaptive traits at both poles of all five domains of the FFM. Crego et al. [47] provide an FFM maladaptive trait model that illustrates the presence of maladaptive trait scales at both poles for all five domains. The absence within the DSM-5 trait model of maladaptive variants of agreeableness, conscientiousness, extraversion, and low neuroticism has limited its ability to adequately cover all of the important DSM-IV PDs [48]. It is perhaps also worth noting that FFM maladaptive trait models have typically placed some of the DSM-5 traits within different locations than provided by the DSM-5 AMPD (e.g., depressivity within neuroticism rather than detachment, and suspiciousness within antagonism rather than detachment [17, 24]). Nevertheless, the DSM-5 Criterion B AMPD is well understood to be providing a maladaptive variant of FFM general personality structure [8].

Criterion A: LPF

The principal authors of the LPF [49], as well as others (e.g., [50]), consider the Criterion A self-other impairments to represent something different, if not largely distinct, from maladaptive personality traits. The LPF traces its roots to psychodynamic theory in which PDs are believed to be the result of core deficits in the sense of self and interpersonal relatedness [51]. This is not though the viewpoint of proponents of the FFM (e.g., [52]) or authors of other trait models (e.g., [53]). It is also noteworthy that the DSM-5 AMPD was preceded by three preparatory conferences, none of which included any reference to a need for a self-other deficits domain when defining PD. At all three conferences, the trait model was considered to be comprehensive and sufficient in its coverage of the PDs (i.e., [54–56]).

To the extent that an impaired sense of self reflects a characteristic or consistent expression of the self, it would naturally be considered to be a personality trait. "Personality traits are enduring patterns of perceiving, relating to, and thinking about the environment and oneself" [1, p. 647]. A characteristically inaccurate or distorted sense of self is an example of an enduring pattern of perceiving and thinking about oneself. As stated by the authors of Criterion A, "The deficits … are likely to result from processes of temperament, development, and environment that have been shown to influence how an individual typically views himself or herself and others" [49, p. 333]. Indeed, some of the DSM-5 Criterion A impairments and Criterion B traits are virtually identical [57]. For example, there is no meaningful distinction between a "lack of concern for feelings, needs, or suffering of others; lack of remorse after hurting or mistreating another" [1, p. 764] and a "lack of concern for feelings or problems of others; lack of guilt or remorse about the negative or harmful effects of one's actions on others" [1, p. 764]. The former is a Criterion A self-impairment and the latter is a Criterion B trait.

Morey [58], a co-author of the Criterion A deficits, has in fact acknowledged that there is "a substantial saturation of Criterion A impairment in (the) Criterion B constructs" (p. 1197). Of course, from his perspective, this is a problem with how the traits are defined. He suggests that the Criterion A content should be removed from the Criterion B traits. However, this would be removing (for instance) lack of empathy from antagonism or lack of self-directedness from disinhibition, deleting traits from the dimensional trait model.

Psychodynamic constructs have long been accounted for within the FFM. For example, McCrae et al. [59] demonstrated how the 100 items within the psychodynamic California Q-Set are well understood within the FFM. Mullins-Sweatt and Widiger [60] similarly indicated that the items within the Shedler–Westen Assessment Procedure-200 fall within the FFM. The original DSM-5 Section III prototype narratives, which heavily informed the Criterion A deficits, were modeled closely after the SWAP-200 [61].

The Five Factor Borderline Inventory (FFBI [62]), an FFM maladaptive trait measure of borderline PD (BPD), includes a scale for Self-Disturbance (assessing distortions in the sense of self and identity) that has been shown to be a variant of FFM neuroticism. Livesley and Jackson, the former also being an author of the Criterion A deficits, had similarly included a scale for Identity Problems within their historically influential trait measure, the Dimensional Assessment of Personality Pathology-Basic Questionnaire (DAPP-BQ [63]). DAPP-BQ Identity Problems is placed within their trait domain of emotional dysregulation that is closely aligned with FFM neuroticism. Subsequent research has consistently verified the location of these scales as facets of the trait domain of negative affectivity and/or neuroticism (e.g., [64]).

There have also now been a number of studies addressing the question of whether there is a meaningful distinction between Criterion A and B [57, 65]. This research has consistently indicated very large effect size relationships of alternative measures of Criterion A with maladaptive personality traits (e.g., [66]). Some studies have even shown no meaningful incremental validity of Criterion A LPF over Criterion B traits in accounting for PD variance (e.g., [52]), whereas the Criterion B traits routinely obtained considerable incremental validity [65]. Of course, there are also some studies indicating incremental validity of an LPF measure over a maladaptive personality trait (e.g., [67]). However, in these studies the common variance is far, far larger than the unique variance (e.g., [68]).

In addition, incremental validity may not actually address optimally the question of distinctness. If a measure lacks incremental validity, then clearly it is not providing any new, unique information. Incremental validity though is simply indicating that some of the variance within the criterion measure is uniquely accounted for. Maladaptive personality traits have also been shown to obtain incremental validity over normal FFM traits in accounting for PD variance; yet, these traits are still readily understood as falling within the FFM personality structure [4, 11]. Even measures of precisely the same constructs will often obtain incremental validity over one another in accounting for an external validator [69]. Any measure of a construct will typically have at least some unique variance that is specific to that measure. In sum, obtaining incremental validity may not be a strong method for documenting distinctiveness, particularly when the unique variance is quite small relative to the shared variance.

More informative are studies that address whether the deficits and traits can or cannot be understood as falling within a common latent structure. For example, Berghuis et al. [70] submitted to a factor analysis the correlations among the scales of a measure of the FFM (i.e., the NEO PI-R [30]) and measures of Criterion A deficits; more specifically, the General Assessment of Personality Disorders (GAPD) and the Severity Indices for Personality Problems-118 (SIPP-118). The NEO PI-R scales did load substantially on and helped to define six of the seven factors. The interpersonal deficit scales loaded within FFM antagonism and introversion factors, and self-directedness scales loaded with low conscientiousness. Nevertheless, Berghuis et al. [70] still concluded that their results indicated that the Criterion A deficits and the FFM involved "clearly distinct components of personality" [p. 704]. This conclusion was based on the finding that one of the four components of Criterion A, identity disturbance, did separate to form its own factor (ignoring that three of the four did not). Indeed, the Self-Identity factor was not at all defined by any NEO PI-R scales. It was confined instead to 19 scales of self-pathology (15 from the GAPD and 4 from the SIPP-118).

Oltmanns and Widiger [71] though subsequently indicated that the identity disturbance results of Berghuis et al. [70] illustrated the phenomenon of a bloated specific factor. Berghuis et al. had included a large number of scales assessing alternative forms of self-pathology (i.e., 15 from the GAPD and 4 from the SIPP-118). Even if these scales assess components of neuroticism, they would likely correlate much more highly with one another than with other facets of neuroticism, such as angry hostility. If one facet of neuroticism is much more heavily represented by multiple scales relative to the others, the respective scales of that facet will bind together to yield a factor independent of the other facets. Oltmanns and Widiger [71] demonstrated that the self-pathology scales of the GAPD separated from neuroticism when an excessive number were included, but loaded within neuroticism when this facet was not represented disproportionately relative to the other facets of neuroticism, consistent with the research concerning the identity disturbance scales of the FFBI [62] and DAPP-BQ [47, 63].

Bifactor analysis is a structural analysis in which the first factor extracted is a general factor representing what is shared by most or all of the scales. The subsequent specific factors concern remaining variance not shared with the general factor. A bifactor analysis is appealing to those who believe that the general factor concerns the core of PD (e.g., what is common to all PDs) that is also distinct from the remaining PD variance.

For example, Sharp et al. [72] considered the covariation among the diagnostic criteria for the six DSM-IV PDs included within the DSM-5 Section III AMPD. An exploratory bifactor analysis yielded a general factor of personality disorder (g-PD), along with six specific factors. They noted that all the BPD criteria loaded solely on the g-PD. Sharp et al. therefore suggested that the g-PD was a substantive representation of the DSM-5 Section III AMPD Criterion A. "Although we do not yet know the exact nature of the general factor, to stimulate further research, we speculate on some intriguing interpretative possibilities … One answer may lie in Criterion A of the new *DSM-5*-III General Criteria of Personality Disorder" [72, p. 394]. BPD is the only PD that explicitly includes identity deficits within its criterion set. "BPD is unique in that impairment in the ability to maintain and use benign and coherent internal images of self and others are integrated into (this) one disorder" [72, p. 394]. Wright et al. [73] obtained comparable findings and reached the same conclusion.

However, both Sharp et al. [72] and Wright et al. [73] did not appear to appreciate that only one of the nine diagnostic criteria for BPD concerns identity disturbance. The BPD criteria largely defined the g-PD in these two studies, but the BPD criteria also include affective instability, unstable and intense relationships, self-harm, recurrent suicidal behavior, frantic efforts to avoid abandonment, transient paranoid ideation, dissociation, impulsivity (e.g., substance usage, binge eating), and inappropriate intense anger. These additional features also define the g-PD and have little to nothing to do with an impairment in the sense of self.

Oltmanns et al. [74] further demonstrated that the g-PD correlates substantially with the general factors of personality and psychopathology, calling into question the proposal that the g-PD is defined by the LPF self-other deficits. The LPF deficits in identity would not also define what is common to such "Axis I" disorders as schizophrenia, bipolar mood disorder, substance use, and panic disorder, nor would the LPF define what is common to all normal personality traits; yet, the three general factors share a substantial amount of common variance. Oltmanns et al. [74] suggest that the three general factors are not defined by the personality traits, PDs, or "Axis I" disorders, but by the common social-occupational impairments and distress that are secondary to these traits and disorders. It is the level of nonspecific impairment that determines one's relative position on general factors (e.g., level of occupational dysfunction), not the presence of a particular disorder or trait that causes this disfunction (e.g., laxness or perfectionism that results in occupational dysfunction).

One can normally interpret a factor by the items obtaining the highest loadings. In the case of the general factor, however, the highest loading variables will be those that involve the most dysfunction. In the case of the g-PD, this will typically be borderline traits as they are the most impairing relative to the other PDs (e.g., [72, 73]), whereas in the case of the psychopathology general factor, it has been the psychotic symptoms as they are again the most impairing. Psychopathology researchers though have not interpreted the general factor as representing level of psychosis because it is apparent that the other disorders loading on this factor have nothing to do with being psychotic. It is perhaps similarly inaccurate to interpret the g-PD as a BPD factor because the other PDs loading on this factor have little to do with BPD. The prominence of the borderline symptoms on the general factor reflects their higher level of common impairment in occupational and social functioning (as well as distress) rather than the substantive content of these traits that are resulting in this impairment.

Conclusions

In sum, from the perspective of the FFM, both the Criterion A LPF and Criterion B traits are understood to be maladaptive variants of the FFM. The trait model involves all five FFM domains of neuroticism, introversion, openness/unconventionality, antagonism, and low conscientiousness (albeit rigid perfectionism would represent high conscientiousness). The identity self-deficit is understood to be a facet of neuroticism, whereas the self-directedness deficit would also involve aspects of low conscientiousness, empathy aspects of antagonism, and intimacy aspects of introversion (as well as neuroticism).

Acknowledgment

This paper is co-authored by Thomas A. Widiger and Gillian A. McCabe, with no additional individuals or organizations providing substantive contributions.

Disclosure Statement

The authors have no conflicts of interest to declare.

Funding Sources

There were no funding sources for this paper.

Author Contributions

This is a review paper prepared by Thomas A. Widiger and Gillian A. McCabe, both of whom made substantive contributions to the conceptualization and preparation of the manuscript.

References

1 American Psychiatric Association. Diagnostic and Statistical Manual of Mental Disorders. 5th ed. Washington: American Psychiatric Association; 2013.

2 Widiger TA, Gore WL, Crego C, Rojas SL, Oltmanns JR. Five factor model and personality disorder. In: Widiger TA, editor. The Oxford handbook of the five factor model. New York: Oxford University Press; 2017. pp. 449–78.

3 Widiger TA, Trull TJ. Plate tectonics in the classification of personality disorder: shifting to a dimensional model. Am Psychol. 2007 Feb-Mar;62(2):71–83.

4 Clark LA. Assessment and diagnosis of personality disorder: perennial issues and an emerging reconceptualization. Annu Rev Psychol. 2007;58(1):227–57.

5 Widiger TA, editor. The Oxford handbook of the five-factor model. New York: Oxford University Press; 2017.

6 Widiger TA, Crego C. The Five Factor Model of personality structure: an update. World Psychiatry. 2019 Oct;18(3):271–2.

7 Clark LA, Krueger RF. Rationale for a six-domain trait dimensional diagnostic system for personality disorder. Unpublished manuscript, 2010.

8 Livesley J. The DSM-5 personality disorder proposal and future directions in the diagnostic classification of personality disorder. Psychopathology. 2013;46(4):207–16.

9 Miller JD, Lynam DR. Missed opportunities in the DSM-5 Section III personality disorder model: commentary on "personality disorders are the vanguard of the post-DSM-5.0 era". Pers Disord. 2013 Oct;4(4):365–6.

10 Shedler J, Beck A, Fonagy P, Gabbard GO, Gunderson J, Kernberg O, et al. Personality disorders in DSM-5. Am J Psychiatry. 2010 Sep;167(9):1026–8.
11 Krueger RF, Markon KE. The role of the DSM-5 personality trait model in moving toward a quantitative and empirically based approach to classifying personality and psychopathology. Annu Rev Clin Psychol. 2014; 10(1):477–501.
12 De Raad B, Mlačić B. The lexical foundation of the Big Five factor model. In: Widiger TA, editor. The Oxford handbook of the five factor model. New York: Oxford University Press; 2017. pp. 191–216.
13 Livesley WJ. Conceptual and taxonomic issues. In: Livesley WJ, editor. Handbook of personality disorders. Theory, research, and treatment. New York: Guilford; 2001. pp. 3–38.
14 Samuel DB, Widiger TA. A meta-analytic review of the relationships between the five-factor model and DSM-IV-TR personality disorders: a facet level analysis. Clin Psychol Rev. 2008 Dec;28(8):1326–42.
15 Saulsman LM, Page AC. The five-factor model and personality disorder empirical literature: A meta-analytic review. Clin Psychol Rev. 2004 Jan;23(8):1055–85.
16 Crego C, Gore WL, Rojas SL, Widiger TA. The discriminant (and convergent) validity of the Personality Inventory for DSM-5. Pers Disord. 2015 Oct;6(4):321–35.
17 Crego C, Oltmanns JR, Widiger TA. FFMPD scales: comparisons with the FFM, PID-5, and CAT-PD-SF. Psychol Assess. 2018 Jan;30(1): 62–73.
18 De Fruyt F, De Clercq B, De Bolle M, Wille B, Markon K, Krueger RF. General and maladaptive traits in a five-factor framework for DSM-5 in a university student sample. Assessment. 2013 Jun;20(3):295–307.
19 DeYoung CG, Carey BE, Krueger RF, Ross SR. Ten aspects of the Big Five in the Personality Inventory for DSM-5. Pers Disord. 2016 Apr;7(2):113–23.
20 Gore WL, Widiger TA. The DSM-5 dimensional trait model and five-factor models of general personality. J Abnorm Psychol. 2013 Aug;122(3):816–21.
21 Griffin SA, Samuel DB. A closer look at the lower-order structure of the Personality Inventory for DSM-5: comparison with the Five-Factor Model. Pers Disord. 2014 Oct; 5(4):406–12.
22 Quilty LC, Ayearst L, Chmielewski M, Pollock BG, Bagby RM. The psychometric properties of the personality inventory for DSM-5 in an APA DSM-5 field trial sample. Assessment. 2013 Jun;20(3):362–9.
23 Thomas KM, Yalch MM, Krueger RF, Wright AG, Markon KE, Hopwood CJ. The convergent structure of DSM-5 personality trait facets and five-factor model trait domains. Assessment. 2013 Jun;20(3):308–11.
24 Watson D, Stasik SM, Ro E, Clark LA. Integrating normal and pathological personality: relating the DSM-5 trait-dimensional model to general traits of personality. Assessment. 2013 Jun;20(3):312–26.
25 Wright AG, Simms LJ. On the structure of personality disorder traits: conjoint analysis of the CAT-PD, PID-5, and NEO PI-3 trait models. Pers Disord. 2014;5(1):43–54.
26 Zimmermann J, Altenstein D, Krieger T, Holtforth MG, Pretsch J, Alexopoulos J, et al. The structure and correlates of self-reported DSM-5 maladaptive personality traits: findings from two German-speaking samples. J Pers Disord. 2014 Aug;28(4):518–40.
27 Watson D, Clark LA, Chmielewski M. Structures of personality and their relevance to psychopathology: II. Further articulation of a comprehensive unified trait structure. J Pers. 2008 Dec;76(6):1545–86.
28 Widiger TA, Crego C. HiTOP thought disorder, DSM-5 psychoticism, and five factor model openness. J Res Pers. 2019;80:72–7.
29 Costa PT, McCrae RR. Still stable after all these years: Personality as a key to some issues in adulthood and old age. In: Baltes PB, Brim OG, editors. Life span development and behavior. Volume 3. New York: Academic Press; 1980.
30 Costa PT, McCrae RR. Revised NEO Personality Inventory (NEO PI-R) and NEO Five-Factor Inventory (NEO-FFI) professional manual. Odessa (FL): Psychological Assessment Resources; 1992.
31 Coker LA, Samuel DB, Widiger TA. Maladaptive personality functioning within the big five and the five-factor model. J Pers Disord. 2002 Oct;16(5):385–401.
32 Piedmont RL, Sherman MF, Sherman NC, Dy-Liacco GS, Williams JE. Using the five-factor model to identify a new personality disorder domain: the case for experiential permeability. J Pers Soc Psychol. 2009 Jun;96(6): 1245–58.
33 DeYoung CG, Quilty LC, Peterson JB. Between facets and domains: 10 aspects of the Big Five. J Pers Soc Psychol. 2007 Nov;93(5): 880–96.
34 van Kampen D. The 5-Dimensional Personality Test (5DPT): relationships with two lexically based instruments and the validation of the absorption scale. J Pers Assess. 2012;94(1): 92–101.
35 Lee K, Ashton MC. Psychometric Properties of the HEXACO Personality Inventory. Multivariate Behav Res. 2004 Apr;39(2):329–58.
36 Tellegen A, Waller NG. Exploring personality through test construction: Development of the Multidimensional Personality Questionnaire. Unpublished manuscript, Minneapolis, Minnesota, 1987.
37 Tellegen A. Folk concepts and psychological concepts of personality and personality disorder. Psychol Inq. 1993;4(2):122–30.
38 Ashton MC, Lee K. Oddity, schizotypy/dissociation, and personality. J Pers. 2012 Feb; 80(1):113–34.
39 Chmielewski M, Bagby RM, Markon K, Ring AJ, Ryder AG. Openness to experience, intellect, schizotypal personality disorder, and psychoticism: resolving the controversy. J Pers Disord. 2014 Aug;28(4): 483–99.
40 Crego C, Widiger TA. The conceptualization and assessment of schizotypal traits: A comparison of the FFSI and PID-5. J Pers Disord. 2017 Oct;31(5):606–23.
41 Kemp KC, Burgin CR, Raulin ML, Kwapil TR. Using multiple measures of openness to experience to capture positive, negative, and disorganized dimensions of schizotypy. Pers Disord. 2019. [Epub ahead of print] https://doi.org/10.1037/per0000389.
42 Moorman EL, Samuel DB. Representing schizotypal thinking with dimensional traits: A case for the Five Factor Schizotypal Inventory. Psychol Assess. 2018 Jan;30(1): 19–30.
43 Krueger RF, Derringer J, Markon KE, Watson D, Skodol AE. Initial construction of a maladaptive personality trait model and inventory for DSM-5. Psychol Med. 2012 Sep;42(9): 1879–90.
44 Schneider K. Clinical psychopathology. New York: Grune & Stratton; 1959.
45 Edmundson M, Lynam DR, Miller JD, Gore WL, Widiger TA. A five-factor measure of schizotypal personality traits. Assessment. 2011 Sep;18(3):321–34.
46 Goldberg LR, Johnson JA, Eber HW, Hogan R, Ashton MC, Cloninger C, et al. The international personality item pool and the future of public-domain personality measures. J Res Pers. 2006;40(1):84–96.
47 Crego C, Oltmanns JR, Widiger TA. Obtaining and losing the maladaptive bipolarity of the five-factor model. Pers Disord. 2020 Mar; 11(2):119–30.
48 Widiger TA, Crego C. The bipolarity of normal and abnormal personality structure: implications for assessment. Psychol Assess. 2019 Apr;31(4):420–31.
49 Bender DS, Morey LC, Skodol AE. Toward a model for assessing level of personality functioning in DSM-5, part I: a review of theory and methods. J Pers Assess. 2011 Jul;93(4): 332–46.
50 Hopwood CJ. A framework for treating DSM-5 alternative model for personality disorder features. Pers Ment Health. 2018 May;12(2): 107–25.
51 Kernberg OF. Overview and critique of the classification of personality disorders proposed for DSM-V. Swiss Arch Neurol Psychiatr. 2012;163(07):234–8.
52 Few LR, Miller JD, Rothbaum AO, Meller S, Maples J, Terry DP, et al. Examination of the Section III DSM-5 diagnostic system for personality disorders in an outpatient clinical sample. J Abnorm Psychol. 2013 Nov;122(4): 1057–69.
53 Clark LA, Ro E. Three-pronged assessment and diagnosis of personality disorder and its consequences: personality functioning, pathological traits, and psychosocial disability. Pers Disord. 2014 Jan;5(1):55–69.

54 First MB, Bell CB, Cuthbert B, Krystal JH, Malison R, Offord DR, et al. Personality disorders and relational disorders: A research agenda for addressing crucial gaps in DSM. In: Kupfer DJ, First MB, Regier DA, editors. A research agenda for DSM-V. Washington (DC): American Psychiatric Association; 2002. pp. 123–99.

55 Krueger RF, Skodol AE, Livesley WJ, Shrout PE, Huang Y. Synthesizing dimensional and categorical approaches to personality disorders: refining the research agenda for DSM-IV Axis II. In: Helzer JE, Kraemer HC, Krueger RF, Wittchen HU, Sirovatka PJ, Regier DA, editors. Dimensional approaches to diagnostic classification. Refining the research agenda for DSM-V. Washington (DC): American Psychiatric Association; 2008. pp. 85–100.

56 Widiger TA, Simonsen E. Alternative dimensional models of personality disorder: finding a common ground. J Pers Disord. 2005 Apr; 19(2):110–30.

57 Widiger TA, Bach B, Chmielewski M, Clark LA, DeYoung C, Hopwood CJ, et al. Criterion A of the AMPD in HiTOP. J Pers Assess. 2019 Jul-Aug;101(4):345–55.

58 Morey LC. Thoughts on the assessment of the DSM-5 alternative model for personality disorders: comment on Sleep et al. (2019). Psychol Assess. 2019 Oct;31(10):1192–9.

59 McCrae RR, Costa PT, Busch CM. Evaluating comprehensiveness in personality systems: the California Q-Set and the five-factor model. J Pers. 1986;54(2):430–46.

60 Mullins-Sweatt S, Widiger TA. The Shedler and Westen Assessment Procedure from the perspective of general personality structure. J Abnorm Psychol. 2007 Aug;116(3):618–23.

61 Skodol AE. Personality disorders in DSM-5. Annu Rev Clin Psychol. 2012;8(1):317–44.

62 Mullins-Sweatt SN, Edmundson M, Sauer-Zavala S, Lynam DR, Miller JD, Widiger TA. Five-factor measure of borderline personality traits. J Pers Assess. 2012;94(5):475–87.

63 Livesley WJ, Jackson DN. Manual for the Dimensional Assessment of Personality Pathology-Basic Questionnaire. Port Huron (MI): Sigma Press; 2009.

64 Crego C, Widiger TA: The convergent, discriminant, and structural relationship of the DAPP-BQ and SNAP with the ICD-11, DSM-5, and FFM trait models. Psychol Assess. 2020 Jan;32(1):18–28.

65 Zimmermann J, Kerber A, Rek K, Hopwood CJ, Krueger RF. A brief but comprehensive review of research on the Alternative DSM-5 Model for Personality Disorders. Curr Psychiatry Rep. 2019 Aug;21(9):92.

66 Bastiaansen L, De Fruyt F, Rossi G, Schotte C, Hofmans J. Personality disorder dysfunction versus traits: structural and conceptual issues. Pers Disord. 2013 Oct;4(4):293–303.

67 Berghuis H, Kamphuis JH, Verheul R. Specific personality traits and general personality dysfunction as predictors of the presence and severity of personality disorders in a clinical sample. J Pers Assess. 2014;96(4):410–6.

68 Sleep CE, Weiss B, Lynam DR, Miller JD. The DSM-5 Section III personality disorder Criterion A in relation to both pathological and general personality traits. Pers Disord. 2020 May;11(3):202–212.

69 McCabe GA, Widiger TA. A comprehensive comparison of the ICD-11 and DSM-5 section III personality disorder models. Psychol Assess. 2020 Jan;32(1):72–84.

70 Berghuis H, Kamphuis JH, Verheul R. Core features of personality disorder: differentiating general personality dysfunctioning from personality traits. J Pers Disord. 2012 Oct; 26(5):704–16.

71 Oltmanns JR, Widiger TA. Self-pathology, the five-factor model, and bloated specific factors: A cautionary tale. J Abnorm Psychol. 2016 Apr;125(3):423–34.

72 Sharp C, Wright AG, Fowler JC, Frueh BC, Allen JG, Oldham J, et al. The structure of personality pathology: both general ('g') and specific ('s') factors? J Abnorm Psychol. 2015 May;124(2):387–98.

73 Wright AG, Hopwood CJ, Skodol AE, Morey LC. Longitudinal validation of general and specific structural features of personality pathology. J Abnorm Psychol. 2016 Nov;125(8): 1120–34.

74 Oltmanns JR, Smith GT, Oltmanns TF, Widiger TA. General factors of psychopathology, personality, and personality disorder: across domain comparisons. Clin Psychol Sci. 2018 Jul;6(4):581–9.

Review Article

Psychopathology

Psychopathology 2020;53:157–167
DOI: 10.1159/000508539

Received: January 30, 2020
Accepted: May 6, 2020
Published online: July 14, 2020

Moving beyond Ordinary Factor Analysis in Studies of Personality and Personality Disorder: A Computational Modeling Perspective

Nathaniel Haines Theodore P. Beauchaine

Department of Psychology, The Ohio State University, Columbus, OH, USA

Keywords
Personality · Personality disorders · Factor analysis · Bayesian modeling · Computational modeling

Abstract
Almost all forms of psychopathology, including personality disorders, are arrived at through complex interactions among neurobiological vulnerabilities and environmental risk factors across development. Yet despite increasing recognition of etiological complexity, psychopathology research is still dominated by searches for large main effects causes. This derives in part from reliance on traditional inferential methods, including ordinary factor analysis, regression, ANCOVA, and other techniques that use statistical partialing to isolate unique effects. In principle, some of these methods can accommodate etiological complexity, yet as typically applied they are insensitive to interactive *functional dependencies* (modulating effects) among etiological influences. Here, we use our developmental model of antisocial and borderline traits to illustrate challenges faced when modeling complex etiological mechanisms of psychopathology. We then consider how computational models, which are rarely used in the personality disorders literature, remedy some of these challenges when combined with hierarchical Bayesian analysis.

Introduction

Studying interactions among contributing vulnerabilities to and environmental risk factors for psychopathology across development is essential if we wish to understand *etiopathophysiology* – defined as complex ontogenic processes through which psychopathology is shaped and maintained over time [1]. Specifying etiopathophysiology is vital because it provides mechanistic targets for prevention and early intervention. This is particularly important for personality disorders (PDs), which are often difficult to treat once established [2]. Traditionally, however, studies of personality disturbance have been confined to those ages 18 years and older given proscriptions against diagnosing PDs among youth [3]. Thus, our understanding of PD development lags somewhat behind our understanding of many other psychiatric disorders.

Fortunately, this is changing [4]. Research conducted over the past 2 decades shows that PDs can be measured reliably in adolescence [5], that adult PDs are almost always preceded by personality disturbance at younger ages [6], and that neural correlates of at least some PDs emerge well before adulthood [7]. This suggests that continued studies of PD development should be pursued. In our work, we study development of both antisocial PD (ASPD) and borderline PD (BPD), which share common

Theodore P. Beauchaine
Department of Psychology
The Ohio State University, 1835 Neil Avenue
Columbus, OH 43210 (USA)
beauchaine.1@osu.edu

genetic, temperamental, neural, and environmental risk factors/vulnerabilities [6, 8, 9]. Details of our developmental model can be found in papers cited herein. We focus here on limitations of traditional inferential methods – at least as typically applied – for studying complex psychiatric disorders including ASPD and BPD. We then describe how computational approaches offer certain advantages in modeling personality and PD.

Current Models of PD: Strengths and Limitations

The prevailing model of PDs described in the *DSM-5* [3] carries forward a typology that has been revised very little since it first appeared in the *DSM-III* 40 years ago [10]. This explicitly categorical model parses PDs into three clusters: Cluster A (odd, eccentric, e.g., paranoid PD), Cluster B (dramatic, erratic, e.g., ASPD, BPD), and Cluster C (anxious, fearful, e.g., avoidant PD). As reviewed by our group and others, including several contributors to this special issue, this rationally derived, discrete model suffers from significant limitations [6]. For purposes of this article, the most important of such limitations concern validity: neither the DSM clusters nor the PDs within them map onto the well replicated, empirically derived dimensional latent structure of personality instantiated in the Big 5. This is problematic because overwhelming evidence links personality disturbance to extreme expressions of Big 5 dimensions [11, 12]. Poor temporal stability of categorical PD diagnoses and high rates of concurrent comorbidity within and across clusters also raise validity concerns [6, 13].

In response to these and other limitations, newer models of PDs have emerged that map personality disturbance onto a limited number of empirically derived dimensional traits [14]. The most straightforward of these approaches assess Big 5 personality traits and closely related constructs, which can become maladaptive – both alone and in combinations – at their low and high extremes [15, 16]. In contrast to the rational approach to PDs exemplified in the DSM, these models are empirically derived using factor analysis (FA), which reduces vast amounts of data into a single model that parsimoniously characterizes patterns of covariance among indicators of personality and personality disturbance.

A somewhat different approach to assessing and diagnosing PDs is used in the *DSM-5* alternative model for further study [17]. Using this hybrid model, general degree of personality impairment is first assessed in terms of identity, self-direction, empathy, and intimacy (Criterion A). Next, specific pathological personality dysfunction is assessed across 5 *trait domains*, including negative affectivity, detachment, antagonism, disinhibition, and psychoticism (Criterion B). Indicators of trait domains comprise 25 *trait facets* (e.g., hostility, grandiosity, impulsivity). Criteria C through G assess issues of differential diagnosis, stability, and sociocultural environment [18].

Notably, all of the approaches summarized thus far are purely *symptom based*. These models are largely agnostic regarding neurobiological correlates and substrates of personality and PDs. Following a largely separate intellectual tradition are models that link personality traits to neural systems subserving *functional domains* of human behavior (e.g., approach, avoidance, self-regulation). According to such models, individual differences in activity and reactivity of core neural systems implicated in these behavioral functions are expressed in personality. A straightforward example is reinforcement sensitivity theory (RST), which describes how neural systems of approach and avoidance interact to confer behavioral predispositions including temperament and personality [19]. RST specifies how neural mechanisms of approach, expressed behaviorally as trait impulsivity at one functional extreme, interact with neural systems of avoidance, expressed behaviorally as trait anxiety at one functional extreme.

Approaches such as RST offer two major advantages over exclusively symptom-based models. First, they provide *theoretical accounts* of etiopathophysiology, the importance of which is outlined above. Second, when combined with appropriate statistical models, they describe *interactive dependencies* among functional domains of behavior. This refers to situations in which one neural system modulates effects of another on behavior. For example, RST specifies how neural networks subserving trait anxiety dampen behavioral effects of neural networks subserving trait impulsivity [20]. We elaborate on these networks below.

Functional dependencies between neural systems help explain different presentations of externalizing behaviors among children, adolescents, and adults who score equivalently high on trait impulsivity, but low versus high on trait anxiety. Whereas low trait anxiety among those with externalizing disorders is associated with callous-unemotional traits, psychopathy, and especially poor long-term comportment outcomes, high trait anxiety predicts better responses to behavioral treatments, less physical aggression, more positive relationships with peers, and fewer police contacts over time [21, 22].

It is important to note that modulating the effects of neurobiological systems on one another are far more common than once thought [1, 23]. This helps explain why functions of single neural systems shows almost no 1:1 correspondences with behavior, including PDs [24]. Such interactive functional dependencies are not captured well by traditional linear models that assume behavior arises from single main effects [25]. In the sections that follow, we describe: (a) our theory of ASPD and BPD development, which includes functional dependencies among neural systems of approach, avoidance, and self-regulation, and (b) how computational modeling can be used to capture such functional dependencies.

An Ontogenic Process Perspective on PDs

Ontogenesis refers to complex interactions through which biological and environmental influences shape development across the lifespan. Through such processes, biological predispositions can elicit environmental risk exposures through self-selective and evocative effects, and environmental risk exposures can alter neurodevelopment. Our ontogenic process model of ASPD and BPD specifies: (1) neural substrates of trait impulsivity, trait anxiety, and emotion dysregulation; (2) how functional compromises in these neural systems confer vulnerability to psychopathology; and (3) why functional dependencies among these neural systems must be considered to understand etiopathophysiology. Although full articulation of our model is beyond the scope of this article, brief description is warranted. Readers are referred elsewhere for comprehensive accounts [8, 9, 21, 26].

Trait Impulsivity

We define trait impulsivity as a strong preference for immediate over delayed rewards, difficulties inhibiting intemperate behaviors, and failures to consider potential consequences of immediate actions [27]. Such behaviors characterize both ASPD and BPD [9, 21]. Although trait impulsivity is highly heritable [28], it is shaped considerably across development by environmental risk exposures [29]. This helps explain why impulsive young boys who incur adversity are vulnerable to ASPD development in later life [21], and why impulsive girls who incur adversity are vulnerable to BPD development in later life [2]. A corollary of such findings is that, in protective environments, progression of impulsivity to PDs is far less likely [9].

Neurally, trait impulsivity derives in part from low tonic activity and low phasic reactivity of the mesolimbic dopamine (DA) system, including the ventral tegmental area and its feed-forward projections to the striatum [27, 30]. This neural network is often referred to as the "primary reward system" or the "pleasure center" of the brain, and is activated when we engage in or anticipate engaging in appetitive behaviors. Low tonic activity and low phasic reactivity in this system imbue an emotional state characterized by anhedonia and irritability [1, 16]. Anhedonia and irritability are aversive, and therefore motivate reward-seeking, impulsive behaviors, which temporarily upregulate mood [31]. This theory of impulsivity – derived originally from invasive research with animals [32] – is supported by extensive neuroimaging work revealing blunted striatal responding in anticipation of incentives among those with ADHD, ASPD, and borderline traits [30, 33, 34]. Notably, when prescribed at therapeutic doses, methylphenidate and other stimulants increase tonic and phasic neural firing in the mesolimbic DA system, elevate mood by relieving anhedonia and irritability, and reduce impulsive, reward-seeking behaviors [35].

Trait Anxiety

As outlined above, low trait anxiety is a definitional feature of psychopathy and callous-unemotional traits, which are observed among some but not all individuals with ASPD and other externalizing disorders. The complex, interconnected network of brain regions that subserve anxiety, including the hippocampus, periaqueductal gray, medial hypothalamus, amygdala, and broader septohippocampal system were also specified initially through painstaking invasive research with animals [36]. According to RST [19], this network modulates ongoing behaviors when cues in the environment conflict in motivational valence (approach–approach, approach–avoidance, or avoidance–avoidance). Suppressing ongoing behaviors in these situations allows cognitive processes to better arbitrate between risky choices.

We have already described how externalizing children and adolescents who experience anxiety show better long-term outcomes across numerous functional domains than those who experience very little anxiety [21, 22]. Among children with ADHD, anxiety also predicts more deliberative responding on laboratory measures of impulsivity, such as response inhibition [37]. Furthermore, experimental inductions of anxiety attenuate neural responses to reward [38], and comorbid anxiety among externalizing youth is associated with less severe structural compromises in brain regions related to impulsive decision-making [39]. All of these observations suggest interactive functional dependencies between impulsivity and anxiety in affecting behavior.

Psychopathology 2020;53:157–167
DOI: 10.1159/000508539

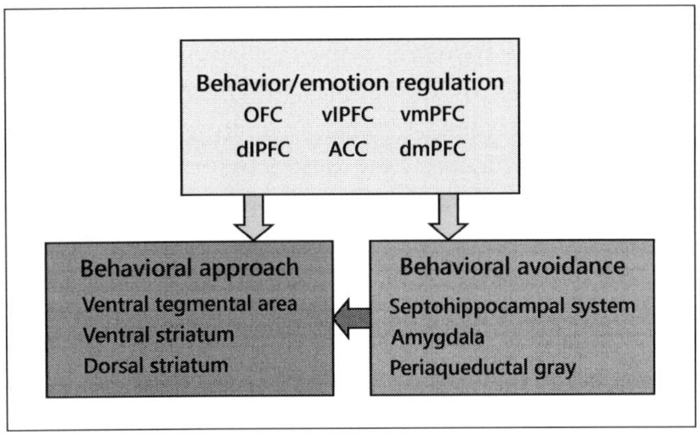

Fig. 1. A heuristic depiction of functional dependencies among neural systems of approach, avoidance, and emotion regulation in affecting impulsive behavior. Impulsivity can arise from excessive approach, deficient avoidance, deficient emotion/self-regulation, or any combination thereof. As a result, disentangling neural sources of impulsivity for any individual may be impossible when assessing behavioral symptoms alone. Furthermore, linear models provide limited insight into such sources. OFC, orbitofrontal cortex; dlPFC, dorsolateral PFC; vlPFC, ventrolateral PFC; ACC, anterior cingulate cortex; vmPFC, ventromedial PFC; dmPFC, dorsomedial PFC.

Emotion Dysregulation

Emotion dysregulation refers to patterns of emotional experience and/or expression that interfere with effective goal-directed behavior [40, 41]. A burgeoning literature links emotion dysregulation to poor top-down control of subcortical neural systems by functional subdivisions of the prefrontal cortex (PFC). Volitional regulation of impulsivity is supported by orbitofrontal and dorsolateral prefrontal inhibition of mesolimbic activity and reactivity, whereas volitional regulation of anxiety is supported by lateral prefrontal inhibition of amygdalar activity and reactivity [42, 43]. Impulse control and anxiety disorders are characterized by disrupted cortical-subcortical connectivity in these respective neural networks [44, 45]. Emotion dysregulation therefore derives at least in part from failures in top-down control over subcortical brain regions that generate approach (e.g., wanting, enthusiasm) and avoidance (e.g., apprehension, worry) emotions [46]. Of note, implicated frontal structures that provide top-down regulation of emotion overlap both structurally and functionally with those that subserve executive function and self-control [47].

Among typically developing children and adolescents, subcortical structures, including the striatum and amygdala, reach adult volumetric maturity by age 5 years, whereas structural development of the PFC continues into early adulthood [48]. Both adults with ASPD and BPD, and adolescents with antisocial and borderline tendencies, exhibit compromised cortical neuromaturation compared with controls [7, 49]. Taken together, the findings summarized in this section suggest that interactive functional dependencies among subcortical neural systems of approach and avoidance, and cortical neural systems of emotion regulation must be considered in specifying the etiopathophysiology of ASPD and BPD [8, 26]. Because these neural systems modulate one another, linear methods that evaluate effects of each neural system, one at a time, on behavior/personality, are limited in their capacity to model pathophysiology [1, 16]. Indeed, impulsivity, an apparently single phenotype, can arise from deficient reward processing, deficient trait anxiety, poor emotion regulation, or any combination thereof (Fig. 1). The specific source or specific sources of impulsivity are therefore difficult if not impossible to infer from confirmatory factor models based on symptoms alone [25, 26].

Limits of Ordinary FA in Modeling Functional Dependencies

Ordinary FA uses simultaneous multiple regression to examine complex patterns of partial correlations between and among manifest indicators (behaviors) and latent constructs (personality traits). Without question, FA has advanced our understanding of PDs, yet as typically applied, it is agnostic regarding complex etiopathophysiological mechanisms of personality and does not accommodate interactive functional dependencies among such mechanisms. Instead, it yields conceptual theories that, although valuable, must be followed by mechanistic research to confirm/disconfirm those theories. In short, ordinary FA tells us which variables sort together; it does tell us why they sort together. It is largely descriptive and therefore of limited explanatory power in isolation [50]. Although additional limitations of FA for making inferences about psychopathology have been described [51], they are not relevant to the argument at hand and are therefore not considered.

Modeling Behavior across Timescales and Levels of Analysis

As outlined above, development of psychopathology – including PDs – is inherently complex [1, 24]. In the sections that follow, we provide a brief, highly focused overview of conceptual and statistical frameworks that more effectively model such complexity across time and

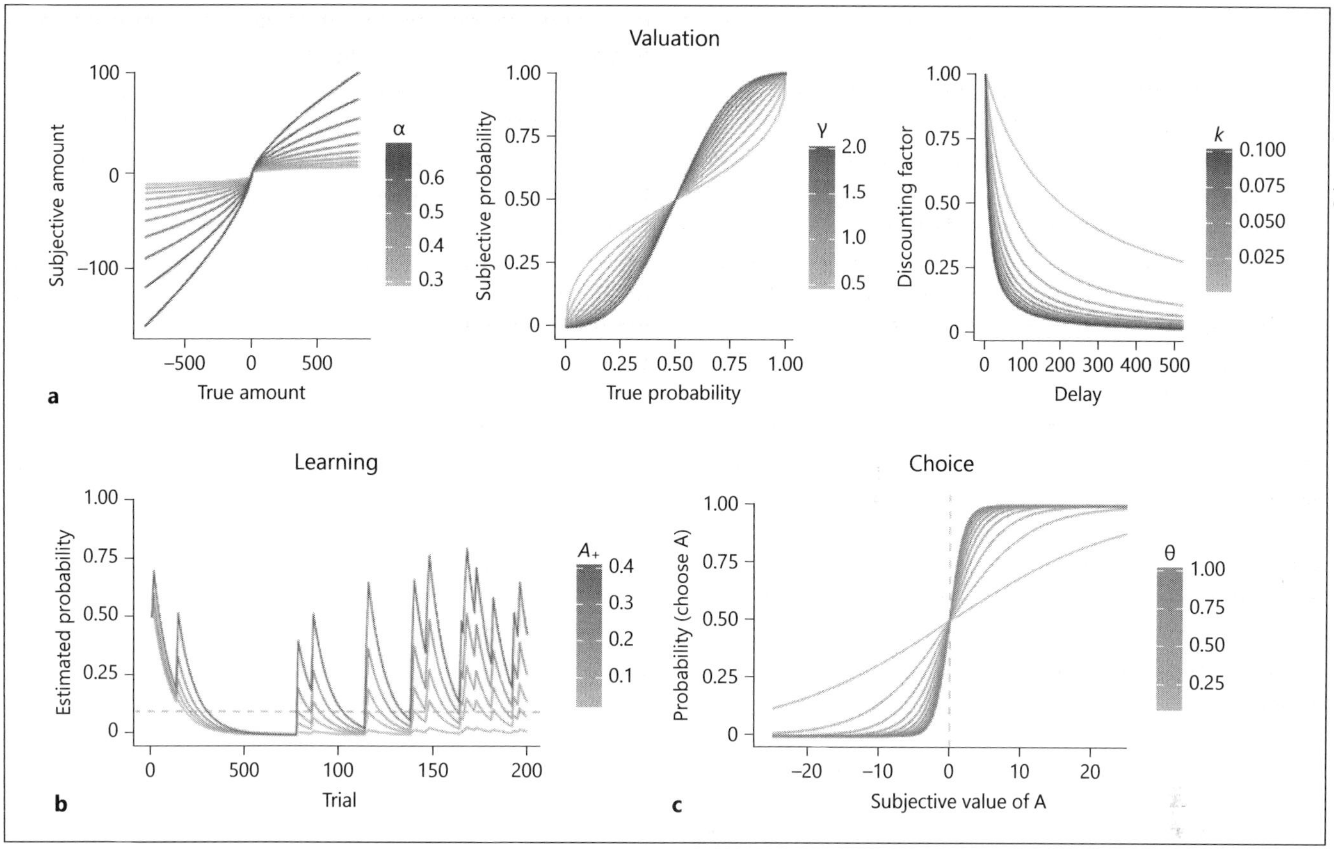

Color version available online

Fig. 2. a Valuation mechanisms offer formal representations that capture how individuals assign subjective value to different dimensions of a given decision. Here, we depict commonly used functions that capture effects of diminishing sensitivity to magnitude (using a prospect theory [81] utility function where α captures reinforcer/punishment sensitivity and λ [loss aversion] is set to 1.5, indicating more sensitivity to losses than gains), probability weighting (using a function that captures overweighting or underweighting of low or high probabilities [82]), and delay discounting of reinforcers/punishments (using a common hyperbolic discounting function [83]). **b** Learning mechanisms can capture changes in behavior over time due to experience. Here, we show learning curves for a model estimating the probability of a rare event (indicated by the dashed gray line, with a true probability of 0.10). The model updates at different rates for positive and negative prediction errors (i.e., when outcomes are better or worse than expected), where the positive learning rate (A_+) is varied and the negative learning rate (A_-) is set to 0.10 in the example [62, 67]. Different learning rates explain systematic over- or underestimation of reinforcer/punishment values (probabilities) – a core aspect of behavioral impulsivity. **c** Choice mechanisms capture how likely individuals are to make specific actions given values assigned to each option/action from previous steps. Here, we use a logistic (softmax) function [65], which shows the probability of choosing option A over option B while varying the subjective value of option A (where the value of option B is always 0, indicated by the dashed gray line) and a choice consistency parameter (θ) that captures how deterministically individuals choose the higher-valued option over the lower-valued option. Together, mechanisms from **a**, **b**, and **c** can be integrated to account for a wide range of both adaptive and maladaptive behaviors.

levels of analysis. Our goal is to introduce readers to these models and their conceptual bases. Given space constraints, we cannot provide full descriptions or tutorials. Interested readers are referred to sources cited herein for more complete descriptions.

Modeling and Identifying Functional Dependencies in Impulsive Decision-Making

Several approaches accommodate modeling multiple interactive determinants of individual-level impulsive behaviors. Many of these approaches overlap despite having different names in the literature. Examples include value-based decision-making/decision theory [52], model-based cognitive neuroscience [53], and computational psychiatry/computational phenotyping [54, 55]. Computational models from these research areas identify distinct contributing mechanisms of behavior, including how individuals represent, valuate, learn from, and choose among actions in response to potential rewards and punishments (non-reward). Individual differences in such predispositions contribute to personality and PD [56].

An often underappreciated but important difference between traditional approaches such as ordinary FA and its extensions [57] versus computational modeling is that confirmatory FA models – at least as typically applied – are agnostic regarding underlying mechanisms of behavior [51]. Instead, they are applied primarily to behavioral data (e.g., self-report items, summary statistics of behavioral measures, etc.) to quantify patterns of covariance among observed variables – with no assumptions regarding the underlying mechanisms of those behaviors [58] (e.g., cognitive, physiological, neural; for a conceptual exception, see Beauchaine and Zisner [26]). Although Bayesian FA exists and can accommodate nested hierarchies, interactions across levels of analysis, and complex nonlinearities [59], it has also been applied agnostically with respect to underlying neural, cognitive, and physiological mechanisms of behavior.

In contrast, the computational models we describe: (a) are based on explicit mathematical functions that model either known or theoretically derived mechanisms of behavior (Fig. 2), (b) can be modified to accommodate iteratively improved understanding of mechanistic parameters (e.g., informed likelihoods), which in turn yields more precise predictions of future behavior, and (c) are evaluated holistically based on how well they explain theoretically relevant patterns in observed data as opposed to whether or not they identify statistically significant effects [60–62]. Taken together, these features demonstrate advantages of computational models toward describing complex psychological phenomena and their underlying substrates. Computational models also gravitate away from the notion that behavior can be explained by a small number of large main effects, toward the more realistic view that behavior is multiply determined by functional interactions among cognitive, neural, emotional, and physiological mechanisms that are often context dependent [25]. We are not suggesting that behavior is subordinate to other levels of analysis in our models. On the contrary – behavior is what we seek to explain and understand. Such an explanation requires us to specify mechanisms through which behavior is effected, across all relevant levels of analysis [2, 6, 21, 62].

Work by our group and others shows that computational models of impulsive behavior, including components described in Figure 2, can: (a) differentiate clinical from non-clinical groups, and (b) generate counterintuitive predictions about behavior based on known interactions among mechanisms [63]. In one of the first studies of this kind, for example, Yechiam et al. [64] used computational modeling to demonstrate that those who show non-specific increases in risky decision-making on the Iowa Gambling Task differ at more mechanistic levels. Chronic cannabis and cocaine users showed a bias for gains over losses and "myopia" for immediate over delayed rewards (higher discounting rates of distant outcomes). In contrast, younger, non-chronic substance users showed no such biases. Similar findings have emerged across a range of behavioral tasks among those with externalizing disorders [65, 66].

Such models hold potential to "bridge" explanatory gaps between behaviors, neural functions, and traits. For example, reinforcement learning models based on DA signaling capture both differential sensitivity to outcomes that are more positive or negative than expected [67], and relations between reinforcer availability and mood stability/lability [68]. Moreover, computational models of self-control link model parameters to neural dynamics, supporting their use as proxies for neural processes that are otherwise unobservable. For example, Turner et al. [69] developed a computational model of delay discounting that includes a within-subject *lateral inhibition* parameter (which functions in the model to downregulate impulsive valuation). When fitting the model to *behavioral data alone*, the lateral inhibition parameter correlated across participants with BOLD signaling in the dorsolateral PFC – a key neural structure implicated in self-control and development of externalizing psychopathology [46, 49].

In our own work, we have shown that trait impulsivity and state anxiety interact to predict delay discounting rates (according to a traditional regression model), and that the same interaction can be produced by a more mechanistic computational model that assumes anxiety and impulsivity relate to distinct decision mechanisms of reward amount and delay valuation, respectively. The model therefore provides insight into functional outcomes among impulsive, externalizing adults with comorbid anxiety symptoms, as described above [63]. These and other findings indicate improved prediction of behavior when theoretical mechanisms and their functional dependencies are modeled directly. They also demonstrate how computational modeling can account for complex interactive mechanisms among individual differences across levels of analysis in affecting phenotypically similar and in some cases indistinguishable behaviors.

Modeling Developmental Change

In the framework described herein, two interrelated types of development must be modeled, including: (1) in-

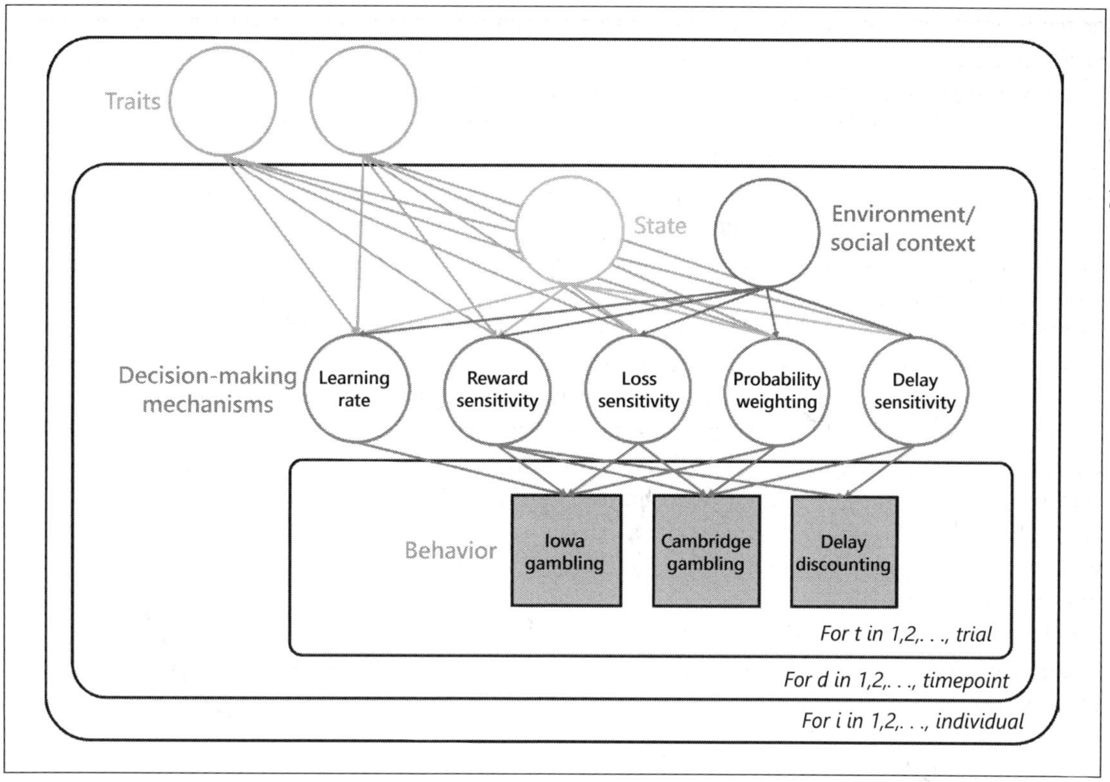

Color version available online

Fig. 3. A simplified graphical representation of how HBA can be used to develop complex models that link levels and timescales of analysis in theoretically motivated ways. Open circles indicate model components with free parameters estimated from data. Gray squares indicate observed behavior (e.g., reaction times to gains vs. losses) in tasks that measure the construct of interest (in this case, tasks often used to measure impulsive behavior). Arrows represent probabilistic relations between variables at different levels. The large rectangles indicate hierarchical nesting (e.g., trials within timepoints within individuals). Note that relations between variables can take any specified form – including simple linear to complex nonlinear. In the model shown, traits such as impulsivity, anxiety, and emotion dysregulation are assumed to exert constant effects on decision-making over time, whereas state influences, as inferred from: (a) physiological, neural, or experimental design data, and/or (b) immediate environmental/social contexts, are assumed to vary across timepoints. Ideally, each level is comprised of a unique sub-model. For example, state effects (turquoise) may be estimated from a general linear model applied to neuroimaging data (red), and traits from FA (green). Such joint modeling methods can improve the precision of parameter estimates at all levels [53]. Similarly, development could be modeled through estimating changes in traits or environmental/social contexts across timepoints, as is often done using growth models. Unlike non-Bayesian methods, prior expert information can be used to constrain estimation at all levels in the form of prior distributions, which can greatly improve the quality of inference (particularly in small samples) [84]. Similarly, once relations are identified, we can use posterior simulations to predict how different trait/state/context effects may affect behavior, which can lead to insightful and sometimes counterintuitive theoretical predictions [63].

dividual-level maturation in behavioral traits, neurobiological functions, and cognitive processes; and (2) environmental-/social-level changes in types and availabilities of reinforcers over time. For individual-level change, developmental computational psychiatry offers a framework that is well suited to bridge behavioral and neural levels of analysis [70]. For example, computational models of reward learning show that prediction error coding in the striatum grows during childhood, peaks in adolescence, and declines in adulthood [71]. Future research might examine how such findings relate to functional changes in neural systems implicated in anxiety and self-regulation, and how functional neuromaturation and dependencies among neural systems relate to development of personality and PDs. Learning models also hold potential for evaluating cognitive and neural mechanisms of treatment response [72]. We note here that latent growth curve models, which extend FA to longitudinal data, could in principle be applied to such data. To date, however, few such applications have appeared in the literature. Nevertheless, joint modeling in which highly precise laboratory response parameters (indexed by computational models), are "linked" to personality attributes over time (indexed using FA), hold considerable promise (Fig. 3). Furthermore, statistical approaches such as hierarchical Bayesian analysis (HBA; described below) offer unified frameworks within which such models can be developed [53, 59].

Borrowing from computational sociology and epidemiology, environmental and social changes are modeled as interactions among networks of individuals (termed "agents") over time [73]. Including these effects is essential given overwhelming evidence that nonshared environments magnify personality traits across development [16]. Using such a framework, complex nested family effects and broader social dynamics can emerge from simple decision mechanisms/rules that individuals follow within immediate, proximal, and more distal social networks [74]. Such models are already used to infer etiological factors of disease spread following chemical exposures, and to identify possible contributing factors to spatially correlated disease expressions [59, 75].

HBA to Link Levels of Analysis

Continuing with this discussion, HBA provides a straightforward statistical framework for developing and estimating parameters from complex models that include individual-level, social, and developmental mechanisms (Fig. 3). A principal benefit of HBA over competing approaches is that it simultaneously pools information across all levels of analysis, which: (a) increases the precision of parameter estimates at each level, and (b) allows us to integrate over uncertainty ("error" in frequentist terms) both within and across levels. More importantly, HBA allows parameters in complex computational models to be estimated simultaneously with parameters from more traditional measurement models in individual differences research [76]. For example, with HBA we can fit: (1) a confirmatory factor analytic model to self-report trait measures, (2) a computational model to precise behavioral data (e.g., reaction times, response latencies, etc.), and (3) estimate relations between individual difference estimates from (1) and (2), i.e., correlations between latent traits and computational model parameters – all within a single model. We cannot provide a detailed description of HBA here. Instead, we refer readers to beginning and advanced tutorials [53, 77–80].

For personality/PDs researchers, use of HBA and computational modeling allows us to ask questions that are more difficult and, in some cases, impossible to address with traditional approaches. For example, once associations between traits and decision mechanisms are identified, we can use these identified estimates to inform prior distributions in future studies using HBA, facilitating accumulation of empirical knowledge and iterating toward more efficient prediction of future behavior. Priors can also be used to simulate effects of changes in traits on future behavior through their influence on decision-making. Because decision mechanisms are shared across many behavioral contexts (e.g., both risky decision-making tasks and delay-discounting tasks require people valuate rewards) and interact in complex yet interpretable ways to affect behavior [53], computational methods are often conducive to more rapid theory development and testing than traditional approaches that seek 1:1 correspondences between traits and behavior.

Discussion

PDs emerge from complex interactions among biological predispositions and environmental risk factors across development. Traditional statistical models such as confirmatory FA are useful in delineating the latent structure of PDs, but tell us little about underlying mechanisms of behavior. This is especially problematic when apparently single behavioral phenotypes derive from multiple, functionally dependent neural processes. As the field moves toward treatments that target mechanisms of psychopathology directly (sometimes termed precision psychiatry), specifying etiopathophysiology at the individual level will be increasingly important. For example, impulsivity that derives exclusively from deficient mesolimbic DA activity/reactivity will likely respond better to stimulants than impulsivity derived exclusively from poor top-down executive control.

PDs and all behavioral traits are determined by complex interactions among genetically influenced personality attributes, neural and physiological organization and activity, physical and psychological states, social and environmental contexts across development [6, 8, 9, 21]. Computational modeling offers a set of methods for interrogating functional dependencies among these complex determinants of behavior, and HBA offers a flexible statistical framework that accommodates such complexity. Although the full promise of computational approaches is yet to be realized, we anticipate rapid progress in the upcoming decades as computational methods become increasingly accessible [77].

Statement of Ethics

No participant data were used for this paper.

Disclosure Statement

The authors declare no conflicts of interest.

Funding Sources

Preparation of this article was supported by grants UH2DE025980 and UL1TR002733 from the National Institutes of Health.

Author Contributions

N.H. and T.P.B drafted the paper. Both authors contributed to the concepts described throughout the paper and approved of the final version.

References

1 Beauchaine TP, Constantino JN. Redefining the endophenotype concept to accommodate transdiagnostic vulnerabilities and etiological complexity. Biomarkers Med. 2017 Sep;11(9):769–80.

2 Beauchaine TP, Hinshaw SP, Bridge JA. Nonsuicidal self-injury and suicidal behaviors in girls: the case for targeted prevention in preadolescence. Clin Psychol Sci. 2019 Jul;7(4):643–67.

3 American Psychiatric Association. Diagnostic and statistical manual of mental disorders. 5th ed. Arlington (VA): APA; 2013.

4 Cicchetti D. Illustrative developmental psychopathology perspectives on precursors and pathways to personality disorder: commentary on the special issue. J Pers Disord. 2014 Feb;28(1):172–9.

5 Miller AL, Muehlenkamp JJ, Jacobson CM. Fact or fiction: diagnosing borderline personality disorder in adolescents. Clin Psychol Rev. 2008 Jul;28(6):969–81.

6 Beauchaine TP, Klein DN, Crowell SE, Derbidge C, Gatzke-Kopp L. Multifinality in the development of personality disorders: a Biology x Sex x Environment interaction model of antisocial and borderline traits. Dev Psychopathol. 2009;21(3):735–70.

7 Beauchaine TP, Sauder CL, Derbidge CM, Uyeji LL. Self-injuring adolescent girls exhibit insular cortex volumetric abnormalities that are similar to those seen in adults with borderline personality disorder. Dev Psychopathol. 2019 Oct;31(4):1203–12.

8 Beauchaine TP. A developmental psychopathology perspective on the emergence of antisocial and borderline personality pathologies across the lifespan. In: Lejuez CW, Gratz KL, editors. Handbook of personality disorders. NY: Cambridge University Press; 2020. pp. 94–8.

9 Crowell SE, Beauchaine TP, Linehan MM. A biosocial developmental model of borderline personality: elaborating and extending Linehan's theory. Psychol Bull. 2009 May;135(3):495–510.

10 American Psychiatric Association. Diagnostic and statistical manual of mental disorders. 3rd ed. Washington: APA; 1980.

11 Krueger RF, Eaton NR, Clark LA, Watson D, Markon KE, Derringer J, et al. Deriving an empirical structure of personality pathology for DSM-5. J Pers Disord. 2011 Apr;25(2):170–91.

12 Trull TJ, Widiger TA. Dimensional models of personality: the five-factor model and the DSM-5. Dialogues Clin Neurosci. 2013 Jun;15(2):135–46.

13 Durbin CE, Klein DN. Ten-year stability of personality disorders among outpatients with mood disorders. J Abnorm Psychol. 2006 Feb;115(1):75–84.

14 Widiger TA, Costa PT, editors. Personality disorders and the five-factor model of personality. 3rd ed. Washington: American Psychological Association; 2013. https://doi.org/10.1037/13939-000.

15 Bagby RM, Widiger TA. Five Factor Model personality disorder scales: an introduction to a special section on assessment of maladaptive variants of the five factor model. Psychol Assess. 2018 Jan;30(1):1–9.

16 Beauchaine TP, Tackett JL. Irritability as a transdiagnostic vulnerability trait: current issues and future directions. Behav Ther. 2020 Mar;51(2):350–64.

17 Zachar P, Krueger RF, Kendler KS. Personality disorder in DSM-5: an oral history. Psychol Med. 2016 Jan;46(1):1–10.

18 Waugh MH, Hopwood CJ, Krueger RF, Morey LC, Pincus AL, Wright AG. Psychological assessment with the DSM-5 alternative model for personality disorders: tradition and innovation. Prof Psychol Res Pr. 2017 Apr;48(2):79–89.

19 Corr PJ, McNaughton N. Neuroscience and approach/avoidance personality traits: a two stage (valuation-motivation) approach. Neurosci Biobehav Rev. 2012 Nov;36(10):2339–54.

20 Corr PJ, McNaughton N. Neural mechanisms of low trait anxiety and risk for externalizing behavior. In: Beauchaine TP, Hinshaw SP, editors. The Oxford handbook of externalizing spectrum disorders. NY: Oxford University Press; 2016. pp. 220–38.

21 Beauchaine TP, Zisner AR, Sauder CL. Trait impulsivity and the externalizing spectrum. Annu Rev Clin Psychol. 2017 May;13(1):343–68.

22 Walker JL, Lahey BB, Russo MF, Frick PJ, Christ MA, McBurnett K, et al. Anxiety, inhibition, and conduct disorder in children: I. Relations to social impairment. J Am Acad Child Adolesc Psychiatry. 1991 Mar;30(2):187–91.

23 Finucane B, Challman TD, Martin CL, Ledbetter DH. Shift happens: family background influences clinical variability in genetic neurodevelopmental disorders. Genet Med. 2016 Apr;18(4):302–4.

24 Beauchaine TP, Constantino JN, Hayden EP. Psychiatry and developmental psychopathology: unifying themes and future directions. Compr Psychiatry. 2018 Nov;87:143–52.

25 Beauchaine TP, Hinshaw SP. RDoC and psychopathology among youth: misplaced assumptions and an agenda for future research. J Clin Child Adolesc Psychol. 2020 June;49(3):322–40.

26 Beauchaine TP, Zisner A. Motivation, emotion regulation, and the latent structure of psychopathology: an integrative and convergent historical perspective. Int J Psychophysiol. 2017 Sep;119:108–18.

27 Sagvolden T, Johansen EB, Aase H, Russell VA. A dynamic developmental theory of attention-deficit/hyperactivity disorder (ADHD) predominantly hyperactive/impulsive and combined subtypes. Behav Brain Sci. 2005;28(3):397–419.

28 Dhamija D, Tuvblad C, Baker LA. Behavioral genetics of the externalizing spectrum. In: Beauchaine TP, Hinshaw SP, editors. The Oxford handbook of externalizing spectrum disorders. NY: Oxford University Press; 2016. pp. 105–24.

29 Burt SA. Rethinking environmental contributions to child and adolescent psychopathology: a meta-analysis of shared environmental influences. Psychol Bull. 2009 Jul;135(4):608–37.

30 Plichta MM, Scheres A. Ventral-striatal responsiveness during reward anticipation in ADHD and its relation to trait impulsivity in the healthy population: a meta-analytic review of the fMRI literature. Neurosci Biobehav Rev. 2014 Jan;38:125–34.

31 Zisner A, Beauchaine TP. Neural substrates of trait impulsivity, anhedonia, and irritability: mechanisms of heterotypic comorbidity between externalizing disorders and unipolar depression. Dev Psychopathol. 2016 Nov; 28(4pt1):1177–208.
32 Milner PM. Brain-stimulation reward: a review. Can J Psychol. 1991 Mar;45(1):1–36.
33 Murray L, Shaw DS, Forbes EE, Hyde LW. Reward-related neural correlates of antisocial behavior and callous–unemotional traits in young men. Biol Psychiatry Cogn Neurosci Neuroimaging. 2017 May;2(4): 346–54.
34 Sauder CL, Derbidge CM, Beauchaine TP. Neural responses to monetary incentives among self-injuring adolescent girls. Dev Psychopathol. 2016 Feb;28(1):277–91.
35 Rubia K, Halari R, Cubillo A, Mohammad AM, Brammer M, Taylor E. Methylphenidate normalises activation and functional connectivity deficits in attention and motivation networks in medication-naïve children with ADHD during a rewarded continuous performance task. Neuropharmacology. 2009 Dec; 57(7-8):640–52.
36 Gray JA, McNaughton N. The neuropsychology of anxiety: An enquiry into the functions of the septo-hippocampal system. 2nd ed. Oxford, UK: Oxford University Press; 2000.
37 Bloemsma JM, Boer F, Arnold R, Banaschewski T, Faraone SV, Buitelaar JK, et al. Comorbid anxiety and neurocognitive dysfunctions in children with ADHD. Eur Child Adolesc Psychiatry. 2013 Apr;22(4):225–34.
38 Engelmann JB, Meyer F, Fehr E, Ruff CC. Anticipatory anxiety disrupts neural valuation during risky choice. J Neurosci. 2015 Feb; 35(7):3085–99.
39 Sauder CL, Beauchaine TP, Gatzke-Kopp LM, Shannon KE, Aylward E. Neuroanatomical correlates of heterotypic comorbidity in externalizing male adolescents. J Clin Child Adolesc Psychol. 2012;41(3):346–52.
40 Beauchaine TP, Cicchetti D. Emotion dysregulation and emerging psychopathology: A transdiagnostic, transdisciplinary perspective. Dev Psychopathol. 2019 Aug;31(3):799–804.
41 Beauchaine TP, Crowell SE, editors. The Oxford handbook of emotion dysregulation. New York: Oxford University Press; 2020. https://doi.org/10.1093/oxfordhb/9780190689285.001.0001.
42 Heatherton TF. Neuroscience of self and self-regulation. Annu Rev Psychol. 2011;62(1): 363–90.
43 Tone EB, Garn CL, Pine DS. Anxiety regulation: A developmental psychopathology perspective. In: Cicchetti D, editor. Developmental neuroscience. Developmental psychopathology. Volume 2. 3rd ed. Hoboken (NJ): Wiley; 2016. pp. 523–56.
44 Gold AL, Shechner T, Farber MJ, Spiro CN, Leibenluft E, Pine DS, et al. Amygdala-cortical connectivity: associations with anxiety, development, and threat. Depress Anxiety. 2016 Oct;33(10):917–26.
45 Shannon KE, Sauder C, Beauchaine TP, Gatzke-Kopp LM. Disrupted effective connectivity between the medial frontal cortex and the caudate in adolescent boys with externalizing behavior disorders. Crim Justice Behav. 2009; 36(11):1141–57.
46 Beauchaine TP. Future directions in emotion dysregulation and youth psychopathology. J Clin Child Adolesc Psychol. 2015;44(5):875–96.
47 Zelazo PD. Executive function: reflection, iterative reprocessing, complexity, and the developing brain. Dev Rev. 2015;38:55–68.
48 Brain Development Cooperative Group. Total and regional brain volumes in a population-based normative sample from 4 to 18 years: the NIH MRI Study of Normal Brain Development. Cereb Cortex. 2012 Jan;22(1): 1–12.
49 De Brito SA, Mechelli A, Wilke M, Laurens KR, Jones AP, Barker GJ, et al. Size matters: increased grey matter in boys with conduct problems and callous-unemotional traits. Brain. 2009 Apr;132(Pt 4):843–52.
50 McDonough-Caplan H, Klein DN, Beauchaine TP. Comorbidity and continuity of depression and conduct problems from elementary school to adolescence. J Abnorm Psychol. 2018 Apr;127(3):326–37.
51 Burns GL, Geiser C, Servera M, Becker SP, Beauchaine TP. Application of the bifactor S-1 model to multisource ratings of ADHD/ODD symptoms: an appropriate bifactor model for symptom ratings. J Abn Child Psychol. 2020;48(7):881–94.
52 Doya K. Modulators of decision making. Nat Neurosci. 2008 Apr;11(4):410–6.
53 Turner BM, Forstmann BU, Love BC, Palmeri TJ, Van Maanen L. Approaches to analysis in model-based cognitive neuroscience. J Math Psychol. 2017 Feb;76B:65–79.
54 Wiecki TV, Poland J, Frank MJ. Model-based cognitive neuroscience approaches to computational psychiatry: clustering and classification. Clin Psychol Sci. 2015;3(3): 378–99.
55 Patzelt EH, Hartley CA, Gershman SJ. Computational phenotyping: using models to understand individual differences in personality, development, and mental illness. Personal Neurosci. 2018 Oct;1:e18.
56 Hirsh JB, Morisano D, Peterson JB. Delay discounting: interactions between personality and cognitive ability. J Res Pers. 2008;42(6): 1646–50.
57 Bollen KA, Curran PJ. Latent curve models: A structural equation perspective. Hoboken (NJ): Wiley; 2006.
58 Hampson SE. Personality processes: mechanisms by which personality traits “get outside the skin”. Annu Rev Psychol. 2012;63(1):315–39.
59 Ferrari F, Dunson D. Bayesian factor analysis for inference on interactions. J Am Stat Assoc. 2020;1–12.; advance online pub.
60 Navarro DJ. Between the devil and the deep blue sea: tensions between scientific judgement and statistical model selection. Comput Brain Behav. 2019;2(1):28–34.
61 Kellen D. A model hierarchy for psychological science. Comput Brain Behav. 2019;2(3-4):160–5.
62 Wilson RC, Collins AG. Ten simple rules for the computational modeling of behavioral data. eLife. 2019;8:e49547.
63 Haines N, Beauchaine TP, Galdo M et al. Anxiety modulates preference for immediate rewards in trait-impulsive individuals: a hierarchical Bayesian analysis. Clin Psychol Sci. Forthcoming 2020.
64 Yechiam E, Busemeyer JR, Stout JC, Bechara A. Using cognitive models to map relations between neuropsychological disorders and human decision-making deficits. Psychol Sci. 2005 Dec;16(12):973–8.
65 Haines N, Vassileva J, Ahn WY. The outcome-representation learning model: a novel reinforcement learning model of the Iowa Gambling Task. Cogn Sci. 2018 Nov;42(8): 2534–61.
66 Romeu RJ, Haines N, Ahn WY, Busemeyer JR, Vassileva J. A computational model of the Cambridge gambling task with applications to substance use disorders. Drug Alcohol Depend. 2020 Jan;206:107711.
67 Daw ND, Kakade S, Dayan P. Opponent interactions between serotonin and dopamine. Neural Netw. 2002 Jun-Jul;15(4-6): 603–16.
68 Eldar E, Rutledge RB, Dolan RJ, Niv Y. Mood as representation of momentum. Trends Cogn Sci. 2016 Jan;20(1):15–24.
69 Turner BM, Rodriguez CA, Liu Q, Molloy MF, Hoogendijk M, McClure SM. On the neural and mechanistic bases of self-control. Cereb Cortex. 2019 Feb;29(2):732–50.
70 Hauser TU, Will GJ, Dubois M, Dolan RJ. Annual Research Review: developmental computational psychiatry. J Child Psychol Psychiatry. 2019 Apr;60(4):412–26.
71 Cohen JR, Asarnow RF, Sabb FW, Bilder RM, Bookheimer SY, Knowlton BJ, et al. A unique adolescent response to reward prediction errors. Nat Neurosci. 2010 Jun; 13(6):669–71.
72 Moutoussis M, Shahar N, Hauser TU, Dolan RJ. Computation in psychotherapy, or how computational psychiatry can aid learning-based psychological therapies. Comput Psychiatr. 2018 Feb;2:50–73.
73 Macy MW, Willer R. From factors to actors: computational sociology and agent-based modeling. Annu Rev Sociol. 2002;28(1):143–66.
74 McElreath R, Lubell M, Richerson PJ, Waring TM, Baum W, Edsten E, et al. Applying evolutionary models to the laboratory study of social learning. Evol Hum Behav. 2005;26(6): 483–508.
75 Mezzetti M. Bayesian factor analysis for spatially correlated data: application to cancer incidence data in Scotland. Stat Methods Appl. 2012;21(1):49–74.

76 Boehm U, Steingroever H, Wagenmakers EJ. Using Bayesian regression to test hypotheses about relationships between parameters and covariates in cognitive models. Behav Res Methods. 2018 Jun;50(3):1248–69.
77 Ahn WY, Haines N, Zhang L. Revealing neuro-computational mechanisms of reinforcement learning and decision-making with the hBayesDM package. Comput Psychiatr. 2017 Oct;1:24–57.
78 Kruschke JK. Doing Bayesian data analysis. 2nd ed. NY: Academic Press; 2015.
79 McElreath R. Statistical rethinking: A Bayesian course with examples in R and Stan. Boca Raton (FL): CRC Press; 2016.
80 Lee MD, Wagenmakers EJ. Bayesian cognitive modeling. Cambridge: Cambridge University Press; 2013. https://doi.org/10.1017/CBO9781139087759.
81 Kahneman D, Tversky A. Prospect theory: an analysis of decision under risk. Econometrica. 1979;47(2):263–92.
82 Goldstein WM, Einhorn HJ. Expression theory and the preference reversal phenomena. Psychol Rev. 1987;94(2):236–54.
83 Mazur JE. An adjustment procedure for studying delayed reinforcement. In: Commons ML, Mazur JE, Nevin JA, Rachlin H, editors. Quantitative analyses of behavior. Volume 5. Hillsdale: Erlbaum; 1987. pp. 55–73.
84 Schad DJ, Betancourt M, Vasishth S. Toward a principled Bayesian workflow in cognitive science. Psychol Methods. 2020. doi: 10.1037/met0000275.

Research Article

Psychopathology

Psychopathology 2020;53:168–178
DOI: 10.1159/000507377

Received: December 1, 2019
Accepted after revision: March 19, 2020
Published online: May 19, 2020

A Common Metric for Self-Reported Severity of Personality Disorder

Johannes Zimmermann[a] Steffen Müller[a] Bo Bach[b] Joost Hutsebaut[c] Benjamin Hummelen[d] Felix Fischer[e]

[a]Department of Psychology, University of Kassel, Kassel, Germany; [b]Center for Personality Disorder Research, Psychiatric Research Unit, Region Zealand, Slagelse, Denmark; [c]Viersprong Institute for Studies on Personality Disorders Halsteren and Centre of Expertise on Personality Disorders, Utrecht, The Netherlands; [d]Department of Research and Development, Clinic of Mental Health and Addiction, Oslo University Hospital, Oslo, Norway; [e]Department of Psychosomatic Medicine, Center for Internal Medicine and Dermatology, Charité – Universitätsmedizin Berlin, Corporate Member of Freie Universität Berlin, Humboldt-Universität zu Berlin and Berlin Institute of Health, Berlin, Germany

Keywords

Severity · Personality disorder · Personality functioning · Item response theory · Patient-reported outcomes · Bifactor model

Abstract

Introduction: Dimensional models of personality disorders (PD) in the DSM-5 and ICD-11 share a focus on impairments in self and interpersonal functioning to represent the general features and severity of PD. This new perspective has led to the development of numerous measures for assessing individual differences in PD severity. While this improves choices for researchers and practitioners, it also poses the challenge of an increasing lack of standardization. ***Objective:*** The aim of this study is to establish a common metric across 6 widely used self-report measures of PD severity using item response theory models. ***Methods:*** 849 participants completed a survey including the Inventory of Personality Organization – 16-item version (IPO-16), the Level of Personality Functioning Scale – Brief Form 2.0, the Level of Personality Functioning Scale – Self-Report, the Operationalized Psychodynamic Diagnosis – Structure Questionnaire Short Form, the Personality Inventory for DSM-5 – Brief Form Plus and the Standardized Assessment of Severity of Personality Disorder (SASPD). We fitted exploratory multidimensional graded response models and used bifactor rotation to extract a general factor across measures. Factor scores were linked to representative T scores using data from a representative survey of 2,502 participants who completed the IPO-16. ***Results:*** When using bifactor rotation in a 7-factor model, all items loaded positively on the general factor, and the general factor explained 65.5% of the common variance. With the exception of the SASPD, all measures provided highly discriminating items (factor loadings >0.70) for measuring the general factor and reached an acceptable reliability (>0.80) across a wide range of the latent continuum. We constructed a crosswalk table linking total scores of the 6 measures to each other and to representative T scores. ***Conclusions:*** Our results suggest that 6 different self-report measures of the severity of PD capture a strong common factor and can therefore be scaled along a single latent continuum. Our results may facilitate instrument-independent assessment of severity of PD and increase comparability across studies.

karger@karger.com
www.karger.com/psp

Karger

Johannes Zimmermann
Department of Psychology, University of Kassel
Holländische Strasse 36–38
DE–34127 Kassel (Germany)
jz@uni-kassel.de

Introduction

The field of personality disorders (PDs) is currently undergoing a paradigm shift from a categorical to a dimensional approach to the classification of personality pathology. The most prominent examples of this process are the Alternative DSM-5 Model for Personality Disorders (AMPD) [1] and the PD chapter in ICD-11 [2]. Both models focus on impairments in self and interpersonal functioning to represent the general features and severity of PD. This new perspective has led to the development of numerous self-report measures for assessing individual differences in the severity of PD. While this improves choices for researchers and practitioners, it also poses the challenge of an increasing lack of standardization. That is, it is not fully clear whether the available measures assess the same construct and how scores obtained from these measures can be compared. The aim of this study is to establish a common metric across 6 widely used measures of PD severity using item response theory (IRT) models. This may facilitate instrument-independent assessment of the severity of PD and increase comparability across studies.

Severity of PDs

Explicitly considering the severity of PDs in the DSM-5 and ICD-11 is an important step forward for several reasons. First, general severity has been shown to be a strong predictor of current or future functioning [3, 4] and has also proved to be a good clinical tool in treatment planning and implementation [5–8]. Moreover, a general severity factor can account for the high comorbidity among PD diagnoses [9], and individual PD criteria that are central to this factor may inform or replace the general criteria for PD in section II of the DSM-5. It should also be noted that general severity seems to be sensitive to change, as was illustrated by a recent report from the Collaborative Longitudinal Personality Disorders Study [10].

Severity of PD can be conceptualized in different ways [11–13]. Kernberg [14] provided an early and highly influential account of conceptualizing personality pathology according to severity. He suggested that the level of personality organization manifests itself in three functional areas: (1) the integration of one's identity (i.e., the ability to establish nuanced and stable images of the self and others), (2) the maturity of defense mechanisms (i.e., the ability to process threatening internal and external stimuli in an adaptive way) and (3) the integrity of reality testing (i.e., the ability to distinguish between internal and external stimuli and establish contact with a socially shared reality). Kernberg further identified three levels of severity based on the level of impairment in these functional areas, namely neurotic, borderline and psychotic personality organization. More recent psychodynamic conceptualizations of severity (e.g., the Level of Structural Integration Axis of Operationalized Psychodynamic Diagnosis) [15, 16] tend to be similar to Kernberg's model in that they refer to impairments in basic psychological capacities and differentiate among several prototypical levels of functioning [17, 18].

Some aspects of Kernberg's model can also be found in the Level of Personality Functioning Scale (LPFS) [19], representing criterion A in the AMPD. Based on an exhaustive review of 5 psychodynamic measures, Bender et al. [19] concluded that the central feature of PD is the inability to understand and regulate oneself and one's interactions with others. In line with this idea, the LPFS proposes one dimension of generalized severity that is expressed in different areas of personality functioning, namely identity and self-direction (self-functioning) as well as empathy and intimacy (interpersonal functioning). Clinicians are expected to assess the general level of impairment on an ordinal scale ranging from 0 (no or little impairment) to 4 (extreme impairment).

Severity of PD can also be defined by the pervasiveness of personality pathology across different disorders, clusters or trait domains [11, 20]. For example, the AMPD includes a trait model, referred to as criterion B, which includes 25 pathological personality trait facets organized within 5 broad domains (i.e., negative affectivity, detachment, antagonism, disinhibition and psychoticism). This trait model could be used as a measure of severity by simply summing up the number of pathological traits [21]. Accordingly, the official instructions for the Personality Inventory for DSM-5 (PID-5) [22] imply that a high trait score indicates severity in terms of problematic areas for the individual receiving care [1]. Similarly, the ICD-11 classification of PDs infers that the traits are used to describe the personality features that contribute to personality disturbance and that individuals with more severe personality disturbance tend to have a greater number of prominent trait domains [2].

Common Metrics

The shift to dimensional approaches to PD has resulted in the development of various new self-report measures of PD severity [23]. Although this is a necessary and important process that expands researchers' and practitioners' choices, it comes with the drawback of an increasing lack of standardization. The new instruments differ in various ways (e.g., underlying theoretical conceptualizations, emphasis on different aspects of the construct, length and precision, etc.), and one of the main challenges is that data obtained through different measures are hard to compare. For example, measures are available that are based on psychodynamic conceptualizations (e.g., Operationalized Psychodynamic Diagnosis – Structure Questionnaire Short Form [OPD-SQS] [24, 25]; Inventory of Personality Organization [IPO] [26, 27]), AMPD criterion A (LPFS – Brief Form [LPFS-BF] [28]; LPFS – Self-Report [LPFS-SR] [29]), AMPD criterion B (PID-5) [22] and ICD-11 (Standardized Assessment of Severity of Personality Disorder [SASPD] [30]). Despite their semantic similarities [31], it is not clear whether these measures assess the same construct and how scores obtained from these measures can be compared.

In recent years, IRT has been used to develop instrument-independent scales, calibrating different measures of the same outcome on a common metric. By explicitly formulating the relationship between observed item responses and an unobservable, latent variable, one defines the underlying trait and is further able to estimate the level of the latent trait for individual persons (i.e., factor scores or theta estimates) using any subset of items included in the model. Therefore, the level of the latent trait can be estimated using different questionnaires and, ideally, comparable estimates can be obtained. Usually, such models are estimated in large calibration samples, often calibrated to some reference population, and can later be applied in practice using crosswalk tables of sum scores or directly estimating factor scores [32]. This approach has been successfully applied for different self-reported outcomes, including depression [33], distress [34], physical function [35] and fatigue [36]. Using the same approach, legacy measures have been calibrated to the PROMIS scales within the landmark PROSETTA stone project [37, 38]. First validation studies have shown that common metrics can be indeed used to obtain comparable group level scores using different questionnaires [39, 40].

The aim of this study is to establish such a common metric for self-reported severity of PD. To this end, we collected data from 6 widely used measures or their short forms in a German community sample and estimated a joint IRT model to link item responses to an underlying general factor. This may facilitate the instrument-independent assessment of severity of PD and increase comparability across studies.

Materials and Methods

Procedure

Participants were recruited via the survey provider clickworker.de, which allowed for representative sampling in terms of age and gender. After providing informed consent, participants completed a survey that included sociodemographic questions, a brief measure of current symptom distress as well as 6 measures of PD (see below). To ensure data integrity, bogus items were implemented in the survey (e.g., "Please select 'not at all' here"). Participants were automatically excluded from the survey if they answered 2 out of 4 bogus items incorrectly. Participants received 5 EUR as monetary compensation for completing the full survey.

Sample

A total of 924 participants aged 18 or older successfully completed the survey. We excluded 34 participants who took less than 8 min to complete the full survey (less than 2.7 s per questionnaire item) and 5 participants who were identified as careless responders by Mahalanobis distance scores in excess of 3 standard deviations from the sample average. Thirty-six entries were excluded because they were made from the same IP address within a time frame of 3 h, which we deemed indicative of fraudulent software usage.

The final sample consisted of 849 individuals. Their age (mean = 42.6; SD = 16.1; range = 18–82) and gender (50% were female) distributions were roughly representative of the German population (Table 1). Participants aged 21 and younger were oversampled to ensure adequate variance within this age group. The level of education was skewed towards highly educated individuals, with 59.0% having completed an A-level degree, as opposed to 31.9% in the general population. Current symptom distress, assessed by a short form of the Symptom Checklist (SCL-K-9) [41], was more than a standard deviation (d = 1.18) above the population average. Similarly, compared to estimates for the general population in Germany [42], a relatively high number of participants (13.1%) stated that they were currently receiving psychotherapeutic treatment. More detailed information on sample characteristics can be found in online supplementary Table S1 (for all online suppl. material, see www.karger.com/doi/10.1159/000507377).

Measures

Inventory of Personality Organization – 16-Item Version

The IPO-16 [43, 44] is a short form of the IPO [26], which assesses the level of personality organization according to Kernberg [14]. It contains 16 items describing impairments in three domains of functioning: identity, defense and reality testing. Items are presented with a 5-point response scale ranging from 1 ("never true") to 5 ("always true"), with higher scores representing greater levels of personality pathology. In the general population, the internal consistency of the total (average) score was very high (Cronbach's α = 0.91).

Level of Personality Functioning Scale – Brief Form 2.0

The LPFS-BF [28, 45] is a brief self-report questionnaire for assessing criterion A of the AMPD [1]. It consists of 12 items corresponding to the 12 subdomains of the LPFS. Respondents are asked to rate the 12 items on a 4-point Likert scale from 1 ("completely untrue") to 4 ("completely true"). The LPFS-BF items capture both self-functioning and interpersonal functioning to an equal extent. In patient samples, the internal consistency of the total (sum) score was high (Cronbach's α = 0.82).

Table 1. Sample characteristics in comparison to the general population

	Sample		German population	
	male, % (*n*)	female, % (*n*)	male, %	female, %
Age groups				
18–20 years	5.8 (49)	5.8 (49)	2.0	1.8
21–30 years	8.6 (72)	8.4 (71)	7.6	7.0
31–40 years	7.4 (62)	8.9 (75)	7.6	7.3
41–50 years	8.6 (72)	8.9 (75)	8.1	8.0
51–60 years	10.5 (88)	10.7 (90)	9.5	9.5
61–70 years	7.5 (63)	5.5 (46)	6.8	7.3
71+ years	2.1 (18)	1.4 (12)	7.4	10.3
Education				
Did not graduate	0.1 (1)	0.0 (0)	1.8	1.7
General secondary school	4.5 (38)	3.9 (33)	16.5	16.1
Intermediate secondary school	15.3 (129)	16.0 (145)	14.9	17.1
A levels (Abitur/Fachabitur)	30.4 (256)	28.5 (240)	16.9	15.2

Seven participants identified their gender as nonbinary. Population data from Statista – The Statistics Portal and from Demografieportal.

Level of Personality Functioning Scale – Self-Report

The LPFS-SR [29] is a comprehensive self-report measure for assessing criterion A of the AMPD. It captures descriptions of 5 different levels of impairment in the domains of identity, self-direction, empathy and intimacy. It includes 80 items that are rated on 4-point Likert scales ranging from 1 ("totally false, not at all true") to 4 ("very true"). In the present study, we simplified the scoring scheme and used the total (average) score, reverse-coding the 12 items that describe adaptive aspects of personality functioning. In the construction sample, the internal consistency of a weighted sum score was very high (Cronbach's $\alpha = 0.97$), and a principal component analysis of the 4 domain scores provided evidence for a large first component explaining 85.5% of the variance.

Operationalized Psychodynamic Diagnosis – Structure Questionnaire Short Form

The OPD-SQS [25] is a brief self-report questionnaire for assessing impairments in structural capacities, as described in the OPD system [15]. It consists of 12 items that are rated on a 5-point Likert scale ranging from 0 ("not true at all") to 4 ("fully true"). It captures 3 subdomains of personality functioning, including self-perception, interpersonal contact and relationship model. In a sample of psychosomatic out- and inpatients, the internal consistency of the total (sum) score was high (Cronbach's $\alpha = 0.89$), and the general factor explained roughly 70% of the common variance [46].

Personality Inventory for DSM-5 – Brief Form Plus

The PID-5 Brief Form Plus (PID5BF+) [47] is a brief self-report measure for assessing the 6 pathological trait domains described in AMPD criterion B and the ICD-11: negative affectivity, detachment, antagonism/dissociality, disinhibition, anankastia and psychoticism. The 34 items were selected from 17 facet scales of the full PID-5 [22] using ant colony optimization algorithms. Items are rated on a 4-point scale ranging from 0 ("very false or often false") to 3 ("very true or often true"). The internal consistency of the domain scores in 3 large samples was high (mean McDonald's $\omega = 0.81$), and domain scores were substantially positively correlated with each other.

Standardized Assessment of Severity of Personality Disorder

The SASPD [30] is a 9-item self-report measure that provides an index of PD severity. The SASPD is substantially derived from the 8-item Standardized Assessment of Personalty-Abbreviated Scale [48], with the exception of one item covering callousness, which was added to the SASPD. The SASPD is somewhat unusual because it includes 9 items that are rated using 0–3 response options with unique descriptions. The SASPD may be considered an index of severity in terms of PD complexity rather than a unidimensional scale of impairment because it captures 9 distinct and sometimes opposing PD features, which are separately rated in terms of severity. Thus, the internal consistency of the total (sum) score was rather modest in the construction sample (Cronbach's $\alpha = 0.76$).

Symptom Checklist – Short Form

The SCL-K-9 [41] is a brief screening measure for the severity of global psychological distress during the past week. It was constructed by selecting the item with the highest correlation with the total score from each of the 9 scales of the full SCL-90-R [49]. Items are rated on 5-point Likert scales ranging from 0 ("not at all") to 4 ("extremely"). In a representative sample from the general population, the SCL-K-9 appeared to be unidimensional, and the internal consistency of the total (sum) score was high (Cronbach's $\alpha = 0.87$).

Statistical Analyses

We adopted an exploratory approach to determine the underlying structure of the 163 items from 6 PD measures. To this end, we fitted a series of multidimensional IRT models with the "mirt" package [50] in the statistical environment R [51]. In particular, we estimated graded response models [52] assuming a multivariate Gaussian distribution with an increasing number of latent factors,

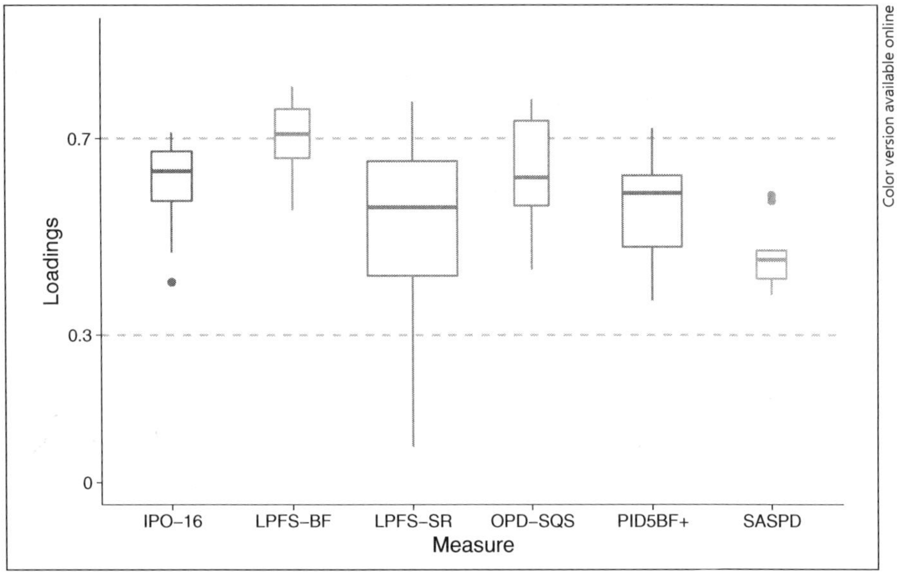

Fig. 1. Box and whisker plots summarizing the factor loadings on the general factor for 6 different measures of PD severity. The lower, middle and upper hinges correspond to the 25th, 50th and 75th percentiles. The upper and lower whiskers extend from the hinges to the largest and smallest values no further than 1.5 × interquartile range.

ranging from 1 to 10. Models were estimated using the quasi-Monte Carlo expectation-maximization algorithm with a total of 5,000 quasi-Monte Carlo integration nodes. The optimal number of factors was selected using the Bayesian information criterion as well as considering evidence from parallel analysis. Model fit was further evaluated using the collapsed M2* statistic [53] and several derivatives, including the root mean square error of approximation (<0.06), the comparative fit index (>0.95) and the standardized root mean square residual (<0.08) [54]. We used bifactor rotation because we assumed a general underlying factor driving most of the differences in item responses and evaluated the strength and reliability of the general factor using explained common variance (>0.60) and omega hierarchical (>0.70) [55].

We then estimated the expected a posteriori factor scores (theta estimates) for each possible total score for each measure [56] to allow easy transformation of total scores to the common metric.[1] Because factor score estimation in multidimensional IRT models is computationally expensive given the exponentially growing number of quadrature points, we fixed the parameters of the specific factors at zero and kept the parameters of the general factor fixed at their estimated value for this purpose (i.e., we used a unidimensional IRT model for score estimation) [36]. The standard errors of the theta estimates were plotted as a function of theta to provide information on the ranges in which measures provide acceptable (>0.80) reliability. We also linked theta estimates to T scores (mean = 50, SD = 10) representing the distribution of PD severity in the general population by estimating the latent mean and variance with fixed item parameters in an additional sample of 2,502 participants who completed the IPO-16 [44]. In order to investigate agreement among the theta estimates based on different measures, we compared these using Bland-Altman plots [57]. Finally, we explored associations between theta estimates and sociodemographic and clinical variables.

Results

Parallel analysis suggested extracting up to 11 factors, the Bayesian information criterion suggested to extract 7 factors (see online suppl. Fig. S1). Further model fit indices confirmed an acceptable fit of the 7-factor model, M2*(11,729) = 23,216.05, $p < 0.001$, root mean square error of approximation = 0.034 (90% confidence interval: 0.033–0.035), comparative fit index = 0.983, standardized root mean square residual = 0.036.

When using bifactor rotation in a 7-factor model, all items loaded positively on the general factor (Fig. 1). The general factor was relatively strong, with 65.5% explained common variance. Moreover, the omega hierarchical was 0.988, indicating that almost the entire variance in total scores can be attributed to a single general factor. Except SASPD, all measures contributed items with very high (>0.70) factor loadings (see online suppl. Tables S2 and S3 for details). The 22 highly discriminating items covered impairments in all 4 DSM-5 domains of functioning (LPFS-SR, 8 items; LPFS-BF, 7 items), as well as problems in self-perception (OPD-SQS, 4 items), identity diffusion (IPO-16, 1 item), and the DSM-5 trait facets anxiousness and anhedonia (PID5BF+, 2 items). The 11 items with rather low factor loadings (<0.30) all came from the LPFS-SR and were often those with positive item content (i.e., reverse-coded). Note that the factor loadings of the general factor had a 0.99 correlation with factor loadings from a one-dimensional IRT model, suggesting that the meaning of the general factor is robust across models with different numbers of factors.

[1] In accordance with previous scoring practice, we used average scores for the IPO-16 and PID5BF+ and sum scores for the LPFS-BF, OPD-SQS and SASPD. To avoid confusion with the original weighted sum score for the LPFS-SR, we also used the average score for this measure.

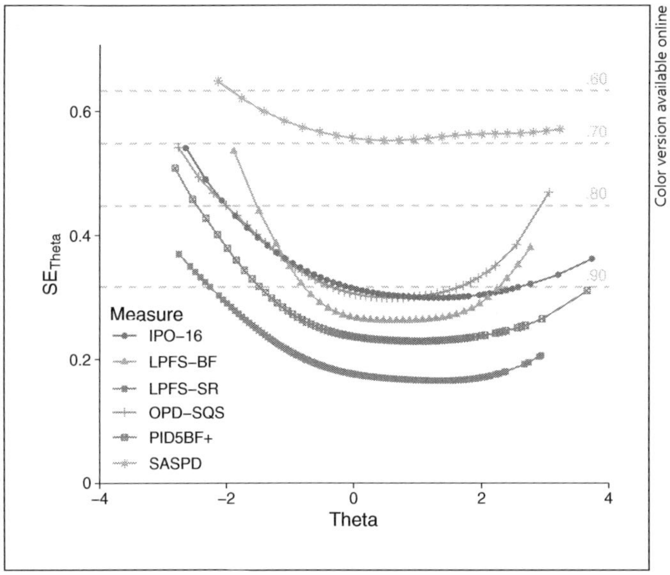

Fig. 2. Standard error of theta estimates as a function of theta for 6 different measures of PD severity. Dotted gray lines indicate corresponding levels of reliability.

Results for the 6 specific factors (SF) suggested the presence of at least two broader stylistic dimensions beyond the general factor. SF2 was defined by 11 items (with absolute loadings >0.40) from various measures capturing the bipolar dimension of fearless egocentrism versus anxiousness, and SF3 captured intimacy problems and social withdrawal (11 items). The remaining 4 SFs are rather weakly saturated, method-specific or difficult to interpret. In particular, SF1 could be interpreted as a method factor capturing mostly LPFS-SR items with positive content (6 items); SF4 contained mostly LPFS-SR items representing impairments in self-direction (5 items); SF6 was defined by LPFS-SR items representing an interdependent self-construal (2 items); and SF5 did not show any substantial loadings at all. Since we were only interested in measuring the general factor, we do not take the SFs any further into account.

Reliability of total scores of all measures was acceptable (>0.80) across a wide range of the latent severity continuum, with the exception of the SASPD (Fig. 2). The highest reliability was achieved by LPFS-SR and PID5BF+, while the reliability of LPFS-BF, IPO-16 and OPD-SQS approached 0.90 at least in the middle range of severity ($0 < \theta < 2$). Reliability was generally lower in the healthier spectrum ($\theta < -1$), and also decreased to some extent in the more severe spectrum ($\theta > 2$). Reliability of the SASPD's total score was consistently below 0.70.

Figure 3 provides a crosswalk between total scores of different measures of PD severity. A theta estimate of 0 corresponded to a T score of 55.7 in the general population, indicating that personality problems were slightly elevated in the current sample.[2] Adopting a normative perspective, an average amount of personality pathology (T = 50) corresponds with the following scores on the 6 measures: IPO-16_{1-5} = 1.69, LPFS-BF_{12-48} = 17, LPFS-SR_{1-4} = 1.66, OPD-SQS_{0-48} = 13, PID5BF+_{0-3} = 0.50 and SASPD_{0-27} = 4. In contrast, a highly elevated severity of PD (T = 70) corresponds with the following scores: IPO-16_{1-5} = 3.56, LPFS-BF_{12-48} = 40, LPFS-SR_{1-4} = 2.90, OPD-SQS_{0-48} = 41, PID5BF+_{0-3} = 1.91 and SASPD_{0-27} = 15. More detailed information on the crosswalk can be found in online supplementary Table S4 and Figure S2.

To help judge the accuracy of the links between the 6 measures, we present Bland-Altman plots in online supplementary Figure S3. The mean of the differences (i.e., bias) in theta estimates between each pair of measures for the full sample was often close to zero and peaked at 0.07 for the comparison of PID5BF+ and OPD-SQS. This suggests that even the largest systematic distortion between two linked questionnaires is less than 7% of a standard deviation in theta estimates. However, the 95% limits of agreement ranged from −1.07 to 1.09 to −1.75 to 1.77, indicating that two estimates of PD severity for the same individual measured using two questionnaires can be spread widely over the continuum. This is, however, at least partly due to the imperfect reliability of the questionnaires and suggests that converting scores in individual cases is associated with considerable uncertainty.

Finally, theta estimates based on all items were not associated with being male, $r = 0$, 95% confidence interval (−0.07, 0.06), or having an A-level degree, $r = -0.04$ (−0.10, 0.03), but were negatively associated with age, $r = -0.29$ (−0.34, −0.21). Moreover, theta estimates were positively associated with lifetime psychotherapy, $r = 0.27$ (0.20, 0.33), and current symptom distress, $r = 0.77$ (0.75, 0.80). The effect sizes (R^2) of the significant associations were slightly lower when using theta estimates from specific measures, with average relative decreases in R^2 ranging from 8.4% for LPFS-SR to 34.6% for SASPD (mean = 18.3%; see online suppl. Fig. S4).

[2] The freely estimated latent mean and variance in the general population sample using the fixed item parameters for the IPO-16 items from the current sample were −0.732 and 1.658, respectively. This means that in the general population, the average level of severity is lower and the variation of severity is larger compared to the current sample. Conversely, the mean and standard deviation of the current sample can be expressed in population-based T scores, with mean = 55.7 and SD = 7.8.

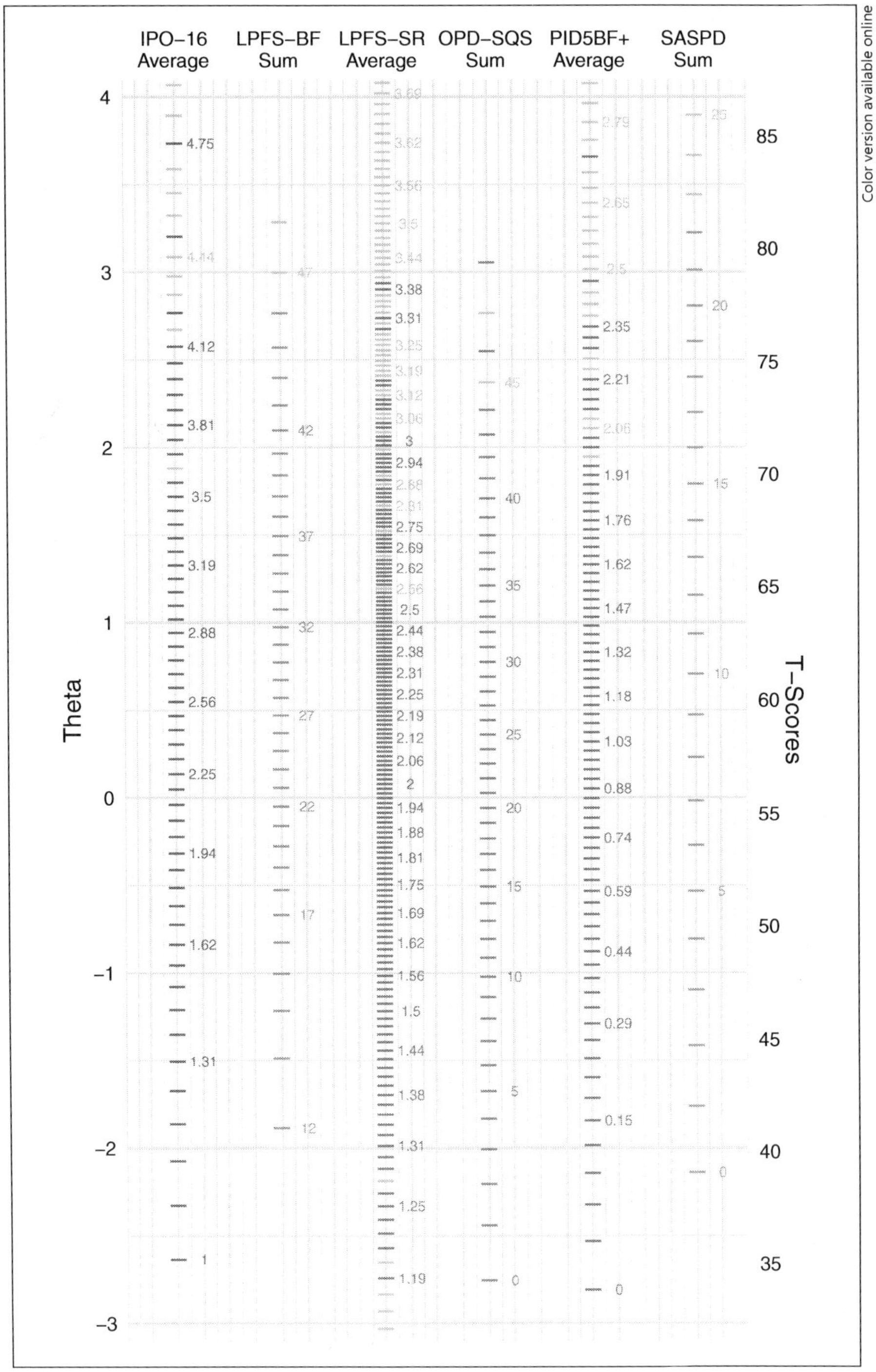

Color version available online

Fig. 3. Crosswalk of total scores between 6 different measures of PD severity. Gray total scores were not observed in this sample.

Discussion/Conclusion

This study aimed to establish a common metric across 6 self-report measures of PD severity. Our results suggest that all instruments assess a strong common factor and can therefore be scaled along a single latent continuum. The general factor was broadly defined by impairments in self- and interpersonal functioning, with a slight preponderance of internalizing personality pathology (e.g., anxiousness, low self-esteem). This suggests that PD severity based upon psychodynamic concepts (IPO-16, OPD-SQS), criterion A (LPFS-SR, LPFS-BF) and criterion B (PID5BF+) of the AMPD and the ICD-11 (SASPD) converge to a large extent when implemented in a self-report format. Thus, our findings extend the family of common metrics to the field of PD assessment [32].

Among the instruments selected, the LPFS-SR provides the most comprehensive assessment of PD severity, including 80 items. Although its factor structure has raised discussions [58], the present study suggests that its large and heterogeneous pool of items reflects a strong general factor. Due to its high precision along the full range of the latent continuum (i.e., healthy to severe), it seems especially suited for individual assessment. The IPO-16, LPFS-BF and OPD-SQS are considerably shorter (12–16 items), but still provide sufficient precision for screening purposes. In contrast, the SASPD seems suboptimal in terms of reliability, which confirms recent findings [59, 60]. One explanation for this may be that the SASPD predominantly captures externalizing and other-related problems (e.g., potential harm to others), whereas the general factor extracted in this study was slightly more saturated with internalizing and self-related problems (see also Bach and Anderson [59]).

Although originally developed to assess pathological trait domains, we found that the PID5BF+ can also be used for assessing severity of PD. This is in line with the ICD-11 model's notion that the pervasiveness or complexity of impairments across different trait domains may be an important indicator of severity [20]. Moreover, this conceptualization is also reflected in the official user instructions for the PID-5 [1], which state that the PID-5 may be used to "track change in the severity of the individual's personality dysfunction over time." From an empirical perspective, this is also consistent with previous findings showing that PID-5 scores align with various measures of functioning [23].

Practical and Theoretical Implications

The study provides tentative norms for each of the 6 measures based on the German general population. For individual cases, practitioners can use the web platform (http://www.common-metrics.org/) to estimate T scores (general PD severity) including 95% confidence intervals based on individual item data. This may inform practitioners as to whether a patient reported elevated (T = 60) or highly elevated (T = 70) personality problems compared to the general population. One advantage of this approach is that missing item responses can be handled more efficiently. Additionally, the common metrics approach provides a crosswalk for converting scores from one measure to another. However, due to considerable uncertainty in individual cases, it is recommended to use this approach mainly for combining whole data sets from studies that applied different measures (e.g., individual participant data meta-analyses [61]).

Conceptually, our results question the assumed distinction between criteria A and B of the AMPD. In line with previous studies showing strong overlap between the two criteria [23], our results suggest that information about the extent of pathological traits may also indicate the general severity of PD. The implications of this finding for a future revision of the classification system are ambiguous: a more conservative conclusion would be that the two criteria reflect the same phenomena from two different clinical perspectives and traditions, both of which are clinically useful and justified. But there are also critical perspectives that find the lack of parsimony problematic: while some scholars argue that criterion A can be dispensed with due to its low incremental validity [e.g., 58], other scholars suggest replacing the pathological personality traits of criterion B with normal personality traits (e.g., the Big Five) in order to better capture the stylistic expression of personality regardless of the severity of the disorder [21, 62]. In any case, our findings support the notion of an "essentially unidimensional" continuum of generalized PD severity, which underlies the initial design of the LPFS [19].

Limitations and Future Directions

We must be transparent about the fact that our results may depend to some extent on our methodological decisions while analyzing the data. For example, we included all items, extracted several factors to achieve good model fit and used bifactor rotation to scale the general factor. A different strategy would be to select a core set of optimal items (e.g., using ant colony optimization) [63], and then integrate the remaining items using linkage techniques [33]. Although we expect that such a procedure would lead to similar results (e.g., when estimating theta), we did not actually test this. Moreover, we used bifactor rotation because we wanted to focus on the general factor. However, it is also possible to use oblique rotation, which may be better suited for assessing the (correlated) pathological trait domains capturing individual differences at a lower level of the hierarchy [22]. Our results do not contradict but are fully consistent with such a perspective. Future studies may also explore the possibility of nonmonotonic item response functions (e.g., generalized graded unfolding models) [64] or nonnormal latent distributions (e.g., semiparametric factor analyses) [65], both of which seem to be plausible candidate models for the severity of PD.

This study provides a proof of concept but is limited in several ways. First, although our sample was fairly representative of the German population in terms of age and gender, the participants were better educated and more psychologically distressed than average. This is typical for samples recruited from online platforms [66, 67] and leads to doubts regarding the generalizability of the findings to the general population. At the same time, compared to clinical and treatment-seeking populations, severe personality pathology was probably underrepresented in our sample, which may have reduced the amount of multidimensionality in item responses [but see 68, 69]. Moreover, the sample size was rather small given the large number of parameters; thus, we were not able to test for differential item functioning (e.g., by age or gender). Future studies refining a common metric approach to PD should include large, representative samples of general and clinical populations from multiple countries.

Second, we only included a somewhat arbitrary selection of PD measures, and several other instruments are available, e.g., the Severity Indices of Personality Problems-118 [70], the General Assessment of Personality Disorder [71] and the DSM-5 Levels of Personality Functioning Questionnaire [72]. Future studies may wish to increase the item pool by combining several samples with different measures and estimating joint IRT models using multiple imputation techniques.

Third, it seems important to investigate the convergent and discriminant validity of a common metric for PD severity. As a preliminary step, we explored associations with sociodemographic and clinical variables and found that effect sizes differed somewhat depending on the measure used. However, across all measures, we found a very high correlation between theta estimates and current symptom distress, suggesting that self-reported PD measures may capture, at least to some extent, rather unspecific complaints or stress reactions caused by current circumstances. Longitudinal studies including measures of constructs that are conceptually distinct from PD are needed to disentangle these sources empirically [e.g., 10].

Fourth, a general concern regarding the assessment of PD severity with self-reports is that typical self-report items can be easily faked. This may not be a great problem in many clinical and research settings, but unsatisfying in (e.g.) forensic contexts. To address this problem, the development of forced-choice assessments that balance the social desirability of response options seems promising [73]. However, even honest respondents may lack insight into some of their behavioral patterns that others may regard as highly maladaptive. This calls for the use of expert ratings [74], informant reports [75] and performance-based measures [76] that may compensate for some of the limitations inherent to the self-report measures of PD severity applied in this study. Thus, a common metrics approach based on self-reports can only support but not replace the comprehensive multimethod assessment of PD that is recommended for clinical practice [12].

Statement of Ethics

This study was conducted ethically in accordance with the World Medical Association Declaration of Helsinki. All participants gave their informed consent to participate in the study.

Disclosure Statement

The authors have no conflicts of interest to declare.

Funding Sources

The data collection for this project was funded by the Institut für Verhaltenstherapie-Ausbildung Hamburg (IVAH) as part of a collaborative project on evaluating instruments for assessing personality pathology. The IVAH did not take part in data preparation, data analyses or manuscript preparation.

Author Contributions

J.Z. conceptualized the study, analyzed the data and drafted and finalized the manuscript, S.M. collected the data and wrote the sample description, F.F. supported the data analyses and critically revised the first draft, and B.H., J.H. and B.B. wrote parts of the introduction and discussion and gave detailed feedback on the first draft.

References

1 American Psychiatric Association. Diagnostic and statistical manual of mental disorders: DSM-5. 5th ed. Arlington (VA): American Psychiatric Association; 2013.
2 World Health Organization. ICD-11 Clinical Descriptions and Diagnostic Guidelines for Mental and Behavioural Disorders. Geneva: World Health Organization; 2019.
3 Hopwood CJ, Malone JC, Ansell EB, Sanislow CA, Grilo CM, McGlashan TH, et al. Personality assessment in DSM-5: empirical support for rating severity, style, and traits. J Pers Disord. 2011 Jun;25(3):305–20.
4 Buer Christensen T, Eikenaes I, Hummelen B, Pedersen G, Nysæter TE, Bender DS, et al. Level of personality functioning as a predictor of psychosocial functioning: concurrent validity of criterion A. Pers Disord. 2020 Mar;11(2):79–90.
5 Hopwood CJ. A framework for treating DSM-5 alternative model for personality disorder features. Pers Ment Health. 2018 May;12(2):107–25.

6 Skodol AE, Morey LC, Bender DS, Oldham JM. The alternative DSM-5 model for personality disorders: a clinical application. Am J Psychiatry. 2015 Jul;172(7):606–13.
7 Bach B, Markon K, Simonsen E, Krueger RF. Clinical utility of the DSM-5 alternative model of personality disorders: six cases from practice. J Psychiatr Pract. 2015 Jan;21(1):3–25.
8 Bateman AW, Gunderson J, Mulder R. Treatment of personality disorder. Lancet. 2015 Feb;385(9969):735–43.
9 Sharp C, Wright AG, Fowler JC, Frueh BC, Allen JG, Oldham J, et al. The structure of personality pathology: both general ('g') and specific ('s') factors? J Abnorm Psychol. 2015 May;124(2):387–98.
10 Wright AG, Hopwood CJ, Skodol AE, Morey LC. Longitudinal validation of general and specific structural features of personality pathology. J Abnorm Psychol. 2016 Nov;125(8): 1120–34.
11 Crawford MJ, Koldobsky N, Mulder R, Tyrer P. Classifying personality disorder according to severity. J Pers Disord. 2011 Jun;25(3):321–30.
12 Hengartner MP, Zimmermann J, Wright AG. Personality pathology. In: Zeigler-Hill V, Shackelford T, editors. The SAGE handbook of personality and individual differences. London: Sage; 2018. Vol III: Applications of personality and individual differences. p. 3–35. https://doi.org/10.4135/9781526451248.n1.
13 Clark LA, Nuzum H, Ro E. Manifestations of personality impairment severity: comorbidity, course/prognosis, psychosocial dysfunction, and 'borderline' personality features. Curr Opin Psychol. 2018 Jun;21:117–21.
14 Kernberg OF. Severe personality disorders. New Haven (CT): Yale University Press; 1984.
15 OPD Task Force. Operationalized Psychodynamic Diagnosis OPD-2: Manual of diagnosis and treatment planning. Cambridge (MA): Hogrefe & Huber; 2008.
16 Zimmermann J, Ehrenthal JC, Cierpka M, Schauenburg H, Doering S, Benecke C. Assessing the level of structural integration using operationalized psychodynamic diagnosis (OPD): implications for DSM-5. J Pers Assess. 2012;94(5):522–32.
17 Westen D, Gabbard GO, Blagov PS. Back to the future: personality structure as a context for psychopathology. In: Krueger RF, Tackett JL, editors. Personality and psychopathology. New York: Guilford Press; 2006. pp. 335–84.
18 Lingiardi V, McWilliams N, editors. Psychodynamic diagnostic manual: PDM-2. New York, London: The Guilford Press; 2017.
19 Bender DS, Morey LC, Skodol AE. Toward a model for assessing level of personality functioning in DSM-5, part I: a review of theory and methods. J Pers Assess. 2011 Jul;93(4): 332–46.
20 Tyrer P, Reed GM, Crawford MJ. Classification, assessment, prevalence, and effect of personality disorder. Lancet. 2015 Feb; 385(9969):717–26.
21 Leising D, Scherbaum S, Packmohr P, Zimmermann J. Substance and evaluation in personality disorder diagnoses. J Pers Disord. 2018 Dec;32(6):766–83.
22 Krueger RF, Derringer J, Markon KE, Watson D, Skodol AE. Initial construction of a maladaptive personality trait model and inventory for DSM-5. Psychol Med. 2012 Sep;42(9): 1879–90.
23 Zimmermann J, Kerber A, Rek K, Hopwood CJ, Krueger RF. A brief but comprehensive review of research on the alternative DSM-5 model for personality disorders. Curr Psychiatry Rep. 2019 Aug;21(9):92.
24 Ehrenthal JC, Dinger U, Horsch L, Komo-Lang M, Klinkerfuss M, Grande T, et al. Der OPD-Strukturfragebogen (OPD-SF): Erste Ergebnisse zu Reliabilität und Validität. Psychother Psychosom Med Psychol. 2012 Jan;62(1):25–32.
25 Ehrenthal JC, Dinger U, Schauenburg H, Horsch L, Dahlbender RW, Gierk B. Entwicklung einer Zwölf-Item-Version des OPD-Strukturfragebogens (OPD-SFK). Z Psychosom Med Psychother. 2015;61(3):262–74.
26 Lenzenweger MF, Clarkin JF, Kernberg OF, Foelsch PA. The Inventory of Personality Organization: psychometric properties, factorial composition, and criterion relations with affect, aggressive dyscontrol, psychosis proneness, and self-domains in a nonclinical sample. Psychol Assess. 2001 Dec;13(4):577–91.
27 Hörz-Sagstetter S, Volkert J, Rentrop M, Benecke C, Gremaud-Heitz DJ, Unterrainer HF, et al. A bifactor model of personality organization. J Pers Assess. Epub 2020 Jan.
28 Weekers LC, Hutsebaut J, Kamphuis JH. The Level of Personality Functioning Scale-Brief Form 2.0: update of a brief instrument for assessing level of personality functioning. Pers Ment Health. 2019 Feb;13(1):3–14.
29 Morey LC. Development and initial evaluation of a self-report form of the DSM-5 Level of Personality Functioning Scale. Psychol Assess. 2017 Oct;29(10):1302–8.
30 Olajide K, Munjiza J, Moran P, O'Connell L, Newton-Howes G, Bassett P, et al. Development and psychometric properties of the Standardized Assessment of Severity of Personality Disorder (SASPD). J Pers Disord. 2018 Feb;32(1):44–56.
31 Waugh MH, McClain CM, Mariotti EC, Mulay AL, DeVore EN, Lenger KA, et al. Comparative content analysis of self-report scales for level of personality functioning. J Pers Assess. Epub 2020 Jan.
32 Fischer HF, Rose M. www.common-metrics.org: a web application to estimate scores from different patient-reported outcome measures on a common scale. BMC Med Res Methodol. 2016 Oct;16(1):142. Available from: www.common-metrics.org
33 Wahl I, Löwe B, Bjorner JB, Fischer F, Langs G, Voderholzer U, et al. Standardization of depression measurement: a common metric was developed for 11 self-report depression measures. J Clin Epidemiol. 2014 Jan;67(1): 73–86.
34 Batterham PJ, Sunderland M, Slade T, Calear AL, Carragher N. Assessing distress in the community: psychometric properties and crosswalk comparison of eight measures of psychological distress. Psychol Med. 2018 Jun;48(8):1316–24.
35 Oude Voshaar MA, Vonkeman HE, Courvoisier D, Finckh A, Gossec L, Leung YY, et al. Towards standardized patient reported physical function outcome reporting: linking ten commonly used questionnaires to a common metric. Qual Life Res. 2019 Jan;28(1):187–97.
36 Friedrich M, Hinz A, Kuhnt S, Schulte T, Rose M, Fischer F. Measuring fatigue in cancer patients: a common metric for six fatigue instruments. Qual Life Res. 2019 Jun;28(6):1615–26.
37 Schalet BD, Revicki DA, Cook KF, Krishnan E, Fries JF, Cella D. Establishing a common metric for physical function: linking the HAQ-DI and SF-36 PF subscale to PROMIS® physical function. J Gen Intern Med. 2015 Oct;30(10):1517–23.
38 Choi SW, Schalet B, Cook KF, Cella D. Establishing a common metric for depressive symptoms: linking the BDI-II, CES-D, and PHQ-9 to PROMIS depression. Psychol Assess. 2014 Jun;26(2):513–27.
39 Liegl G, Wahl I, Berghöfer A, Nolte S, Pieh C, Rose M, et al. Using Patient Health Questionnaire-9 item parameters of a common metric resulted in similar depression scores compared to independent item response theory model reestimation. J Clin Epidemiol. 2016 Mar;71:25–34.
40 Sunderland M, Batterham P, Calear A, Carragher N. Validity of the PROMIS depression and anxiety common metrics in an online sample of Australian adults. Qual Life Res. 2018 Sep;27(9):2453–8.
41 Petrowski K, Schmalbach B, Kliem S, Hinz A, Brähler E. Symptom-Checklist-K-9: norm values and factorial structure in a representative German sample. PLoS One. 2019 Apr; 14(4):e0213490.
42 Larisch A, Heuft G, Engbrink S, Brähler E, Herzog W, Kruse J. Behandlung psychischer und psychosomatischer Beschwerden – Inanspruchnahme, Erwartungen und Kenntnisse der Allgemeinbevölkerung in Deutschland. Z Psychosom Med Psychother. 2013; 59(2):153–69.
43 Zimmermann J, Benecke C, Hörz S, Rentrop M, Peham D, Bock A, et al. Validierung einer deutschsprachigen 16-Item-Version des Inventars der Persönlichkeitsorganisation (IPO-16). Diagnostica. 2013;59(1):3–16.
44 Zimmermann J, Benecke C, Hörz-Sagstetter S, Dammann G. Normierung der deutschsprachigen 16-Item-Version des Inventars der Persönlichkeitsorganisation (IPO-16). Z Psychosom Med Psychother. 2015;61(1):5–18.
45 Hutsebaut J, Feenstra DJ, Kamphuis JH. Development and preliminary psychometric evaluation of a brief self-report questionnaire for the assessment of the DSM-5 Level of Personality Functioning Scale: The LPFS Brief Form (LPFS-BF). Pers Disord. 2016 Apr;7(2): 192–7.

46 Obbarius A, Obbarius N, Fischer F, Liegl G, Rose M. Evaluation der Faktorenstruktur und Konstruktvalidität der 12-Item-Kurzversion des OPD-Strukturfragebogens (OPD-SFK) an psychosomatischen Patienten. Psychother Psychosom Med Psychol. 2019 Jan;69(1):38–48.
47 Kerber A, Schultze M, Müller S, Rühling RM, Wright AGC, Spitzer C, et al. Development of a short and ICD-11 compatible measure for DSM-5 maladaptive personality traits using ant colony optimization algorithms. Submitted for publication. 2019. DOI: 10.31234/osf.io/rsw54.
48 Moran P, Leese M, Lee T, Walters P, Thornicroft G, Mann A. Standardised Assessment of Personality - Abbreviated Scale (SAPAS): preliminary validation of a brief screen for personality disorder. Br J Psychiatry. 2003 Sep;183(3):228–32.
49 Derogatis LR. Symptom Checklist 90, R-Version manual I: scoring, administration, and procedures for the SCL-90. Baltimore (MD): Johns Hopkins Press; 1977.
50 Chalmers RP. mirt: a multidimensional item response theory package for the R environment. J Stat Softw. 2012;48(6):1–29.
51 R Core Team. R: A language and environment for statistical computing. Vienna, Austria: R Foundation for Statistical Computing; 2016.
52 Samejima F. Estimation of latent ability using a response pattern of graded scores. Psychometrika Monogr Suppl. 1969;34 S1:100–14.
53 Cai L, Hansen M. Limited-information goodness-of-fit testing of hierarchical item factor models. Br J Math Stat Psychol. 2013 May;66(2):245–76.
54 Hu L, Bentler PM. Cutoff criteria for fit indexes in covariance structure analysis: conventional criteria versus new alternatives. Struct Equ Modeling. 1999;6(1):1–55.
55 Reise SP, Scheines R, Widaman KF, Haviland MG. Multidimensionality and structural coefficient bias in structural equation modeling. Educ Psychol Meas. 2013;73(1):5–26.
56 Thissen D, Pommerich M, Billeaud K, Williams VS. Item response theory for scores on tests including polytomous items with ordered responses. Appl Psychol Meas. 1995;19(1):39–49.
57 Bland JM, Altman DG. Comparing methods of measurement: why plotting difference against standard method is misleading. Lancet. 1995 Oct;346(8982):1085–7.
58 Sleep CE, Lynam DR, Widiger TA, Crowe ML, Miller JD. An evaluation of DSM-5 section III personality disorder criterion A (impairment) in accounting for psychopathology. Psychol Assess. 2019 Oct;31(10):1181–91.
59 Bach B, Anderson JL. Patient-reported ICD-11 personality disorder severity and DSM-5 level of personality functioning. J Pers Disord. Epub 2018 Sep.
60 Rek K, Thielmann I, Henkel M, Crawford M, Piccirilli L, Graff A, et al. A psychometric evaluation of the Standardized Assessment of Severity of Personality Disorder (SASPD) in clinical and non-clinical German samples. Submitted for publication. 2019. DOI: 10.31234/osf.io/unqhm.
61 Ebert DD, Buntrock C, Reins JA, Zimmermann J, Cuijpers P. Efficacy and moderators of psychological interventions in treating subclinical symptoms of depression and preventing major depressive disorder onsets: protocol for an individual patient data meta-analysis of randomised controlled trials. BMJ Open. 2018 Mar;8(3):e018582.
62 Morey LC, Good EW, Hopwood CJ. Global personality dysfunction and the relationship of pathological and normal trait domains in the DSM-5 Alternative Model for Personality Disorders. Submitted for publication. 2020.
63 Schroeders U, Wilhelm O, Olaru G. Metaheuristics in short scale construction: ant colony optimization and genetic algorithm. PLoS One. 2016 Nov;11(11):e0167110.
64 Zimmermann J, Böhnke JR, Eschstruth R, Mathews A, Wenzel K, Leising D. The latent structure of personality functioning: investigating criterion A from the alternative model for personality disorders in DSM-5. J Abnorm Psychol. 2015 Aug;124(3):532–48.
65 Wendt LP, Wright AG, Pilkonis PA, Nolte T, Fonagy P, Montague PR, et al. The latent structure of interpersonal problems: validity of dimensional, categorical, and hybrid models. J Abnorm Psychol. 2019 Nov;128(8):823–39.
66 Ophir Y, Sisso I, Asterhan CS, Tikochinski R, Reichart R. The turker blues: hidden factors behind increased depression rates among Amazon's Mechanical Turkers. Clin Psychol Sci. 2020;8(1):65–83.
67 Shapiro DN, Chandler J, Mueller PA. Using Mechanical Turk to study clinical populations. Clin Psychol Sci. 2013;1(2):213–20.
68 O'Connor BP. The search for dimensional structure differences between normality and abnormality: a statistical review of published data on personality and psychopathology. J Pers Soc Psychol. 2002 Oct;83(4):962–82.
69 Bach B, Sellbom M, Simonsen E. Personality inventory for DSM-5 (PID-5) in clinical versus nonclinical individuals: generalizability of psychometric features. Assessment. 2018 Oct;25(7):815–25.
70 Verheul R, Andrea H, Berghout CC, Dolan C, Busschbach JJ, van der Kroft PJ, et al. Severity Indices of Personality Problems (SIPP-118): development, factor structure, reliability, and validity. Psychol Assess. 2008 Mar;20(1):23–34.
71 Livesley WJ. General Assessment of Personality Disorder (GAPD). Vancouver (BC): Department of Psychiatry, University of British Columbia; 2006.
72 Huprich SK, Nelson SM, Meehan KB, Siefert CJ, Haggerty G, Sexton J, et al. Introduction of the DSM-5 levels of Personality Functioning Questionnaire. Pers Disord. 2018 Nov;9(6):553–63.
73 Guenole N, Brown AA, Cooper AJ. Forced-choice assessment of work-related maladaptive personality traits: preliminary evidence from an application of Thurstonian item response modeling. Assessment. 2018 Jun;25(4):513–26.
74 Westen D, Weinberger J. When clinical description becomes statistical prediction. Am Psychol. 2004 Oct;59(7):595–613.
75 Oltmanns TF, Turkheimer E. Person perception and personality pathology. Curr Dir Psychol Sci. 2009 Jan;18(1):32–6.
76 Bornstein RF. Toward a process-focused model of test score validity: improving psychological assessment in science and practice. Psychol Assess. 2011 Jun;23(2):532–44.

Research Article

Psychopathology

Psychopathology 2020;53:179–188
DOI: 10.1159/000507589

Received: December 13, 2019
Accepted: March 27, 2020
Published online: May 5, 2020

International Assessment of DSM-5 and ICD-11 Personality Disorder Traits: Toward a Common Nosology in DSM-5.1

Bo Bach[a] André Kerber[b] Anton Aluja[c] Tim Bastiaens[d] Jared W. Keeley[e] Laurence Claes[f, t] Andrea Fossati[g] Fernando Gutierrez[h] Sérgio E.S. Oliveira[i] Rute Pires[j] Karel D. Riegel[k] Jean-Pierre Rolland[l] Isabelle Roskam[m] Martin Sellbom[n] Antonella Somma[g] Lucas Spanemberg[o] Włodzimierz Strus[p] Jens C. Thimm[q] Aidan G.C. Wright[r] Johannes Zimmermann[s]

[a]Center for Personality Disorder Research, Psychiatric Research Unit, Region Zealand, Slagelse, Denmark; [b]Department of Psychology, Freie Universität Berlin, Berlin, Germany; [c]Lleida Institute for Biomedical Research, University of Lleida, Catalonia, Spain; [d]University Psychiatric Centre, Katholieke Universiteit Leuven, Leuven, Belgium; [e]Psychology Department, Virginia Commonwealth University, Richmond, VA, USA; [f]Faculty of Medicine and Health Sciences, University of Antwerp, Leuven, Belgium; [g]Faculty of Psychology, Vita-Salute San Raffaele University, Milan, Italy; [h]Hospital Clinic of Barcelona, Barcelona, Spain; [i]Institute of Psychology, University of Brasília (UnB), Brasília, Brazil; [j]CICPSI, Faculdade de Psicologia, Universidade de Lisboa, Lisbon, Portugal; [k]Department of Addictology, 1st Faculty of Medicine, Charles University of Prague, General University Hospital of Prague, Prague, Czech Republic; [l]STAPS, University Paris-Nanterre, Paris, France; [m]Psychological Sciences Research Institute, Université Catholique de Louvain (UCLouvain), Louvain-la-Neuve, Belgium; [n]Department of Psychology, University of Otago, Dunedin, New Zealand; [o]Escola de Medicina, Pontifícia Universidade Católica do Rio Grande do Sul (PUCRS), Porto Alegre, Brazil; [p]Institute of Psychology, Cardinal Stefan Wyszyński University, Warsaw, Poland; [q]Department of Psychology, The Arctic University of Norway (UiT), Tromsoe, Norway; [r]Department of Psychology, University of Pittsburgh, Pittsburgh, PA, USA; [s]Department of Psychology, University of Kassel, Kassel, Germany; [t]Faculty of Psychology and Educational Sciences, Katholieke Universiteit Leuven, Leuven, Belgium

Keywords

ICD-11 · DSM-5.1 · Personality disorder classification · Trait · Diagnosis

Abstract

Introduction: The DSM-5 Alternative Model of Personality Disorders (AMPD) and the ICD-11 classification of personality disorders (PD) are largely commensurate and, when combined, they delineate 6 trait domains: negative affectivity, detachment, antagonism/dissociality, disinhibition, anankastia, and psychoticism. ***Objective:*** The present study evaluated the international validity of a brief 36-item patient-report measure that portrays all 6 domains simultaneously including 18 primary subfacets. ***Methods:*** We developed and employed a modified version of the Personality Inventory for DSM-5 – Brief Form Plus (PID5BF+). A total of 16,327 individuals were included, 2,347 of whom were patients. The expected 6-factor structure of facets was initially investigated in samples from Denmark ($n = 584$), Germany ($n = 1,271$), and the USA ($n = 605$) and subsequently replicated in both patient- and community samples from Italy, France, Switzerland, Belgium, Norway, Portugal, Spain, Poland, Czech Republic, the USA, and Brazil. Associations with interview-rated

karger@karger.com
www.karger.com/psp

Karger

Bo Bach, PhD
Center for Personality Disorder Research, Psychiatric Research Unit, Region Zealand
Psychiatric Hospital Slagelse, Faelledvej 6, Building 3, 4th floor
DK-4200 Slagelse (Denmark)
bobachsayad@gmail.com

DSM-5 PD categories were also investigated. ***Results:*** Findings generally supported the empirical soundness and international robustness of the 6 domains including meaningful associations with familiar interview-rated PD types. ***Conclusions:*** The modified PID5BF+ may be employed internationally by clinicians and researchers for brief and reliable assessment of the 6 combined DSM-5 and ICD-11 domains, including 18 primary subfacets. This 6-domain framework may inform a future nosology for DSM-5.1 that is more reasonably aligned with the authoritative ICD-11 codes than the current DSM-5 AMPD model. The 36-item modified PID5BF+ scoring key is provided in online supplementary Appendix A see www.karger.com/doi/10.1159/000507589 (for all online suppl. material).

Introduction

More than 1 out of 10 individuals in Western societies [1] and at least half of psychiatric outpatients [2] meet the diagnostic requirements for a personality disorder (PD), which is a central predictor of psychosocial impairment, comorbidity, and treatment outcomes [3]. However, scientific and clinical attention to PD varies from country to country due to culture, zeitgeist, and politics[1] [4]. In many countries, PD are rarely diagnosed or described at all, apparently because practitioners find them too complicated and cumbersome to assess [5]. For such reasons, it seems imperative to introduce an internationally robust and feasible assessment framework that delineates the phenotypic variation in the expression of PD according to upcoming empirical nosology.

In both the ICD-11 classification of PD and the DSM-5 Alternative Model of Personality Disorders (AMPD), Section III, trait domains are used as specifiers that contribute to the individual expression of personality disturbance in addition to the overall classification of severity (e.g., mild, moderate, or severe) [6, 7]. Such specifiers are not diagnostic entities per se, but they may inform the clinical management of those patients who have been diagnosed with a PD or personality difficulty, including how to establish a therapeutic alliance and decide on the target of the intervention [8]. Both ICD-11 and DSM-5 AMPD describe trait domains of negative affectivity, detachment, antagonism/dissociality, and disinhibition. In addition, the DSM-5 AMPD also includes a separate domain of psychoticism, whereas the ICD-11 includes a separate domain of anankastia.

In the present paper, we perceive 3 potential shortcomings of the DSM-5 AMPD and ICD-11 trait models[2], respectively. First, the ICD-11 PD classification remains consistent with the ICD-10 tradition where schizotypy is understood as a variant of schizophrenia rather than a PD. For that reason, a domain of psychoticism is not included in the ICD-11 model. Nevertheless, a growing body of research and clinical knowledge suggest that trait features of schizotypy and psychoticism (e.g., oddity, thought disorder, and schizophrenia proneness) should not be ignored [9, 10]. Second, the ICD-11 trait domain of Anankastia corresponds to the compulsivity trait domain, which was originally proposed as a separate domain for the DSM-5 trait model [11]. Ultimately this domain was omitted in the DSM-5 AMPD in favor of parsimony [12]. The DSM-5 AMPD defines features of anankastia/compulsivity (e.g., rigid perfectionism) in terms of low disinhibition, which is somewhat supported by empirical evidence [13, 14]. Third, another difference between the DSM-5 AMPD trait model and the ICD-11 trait model is that the latter does not include any specific facets within the broader domains (e.g., grandiosity, deceitfulness, and manipulativeness within the domain of antagonism). Taken together, we propose that the aforementioned 3 potential shortcomings might be addressed using a combined assessment framework that operationalizes all 6 domains (including separate domains of psychoticism and anankastia) along with 3 primary facet level features for each domain. It might be worthwhile to consider such a common 6-factor framework in the progress toward DSM-5.1.

A Feasible Approach to Measuring ICD-11 and DSM-5 Trait Domains and Facets

Initially, the 220-item Personality Inventory for DSM-5 (PID-5) was constructed to operationalize the DSM-5 AMPD trait model [12]. So far, several forms and scales have been developed from this PID-5 item-pool, including abbreviated forms [15, 16] and an algorithm for capturing 5 ICD-11 trait domains [17, 18] with 16 DSM-5 trait facets. Most recently an algorithm was developed for assessment of the combined DSM-5 AMPD and ICD-11

[1] For example, so-called "dangerous" PD have received much attention in the UK due to a political and public awareness of their potential risk to others [59], whereas in Norway avoidant PD have been extensively described and investigated for years due to their perceived importance in this particular region [60].

[2] The present study only focused on the trait domain qualifiers. An optional borderline pattern qualifier was included in the ICD-11 to enhance clinical utility in terms of continuity with the well-established treatment guidelines for this disorder, and it may optionally be used after first having specified prominent trait qualifiers.

trait model by means of 6 distinct domains (i.e., negative affectivity, detachment, antagonism, disinhibition, anankastia, and psychoticism), including 17 lower-order facets with a total of 34 items. It is the Personality Inventory for DSM-5 – Brief Form Plus (PID5BF+) [19]. In the present study we developed and employed a modified 36-item version of the PID5BF+, which is further described in Materials and Methods.

Goal of the Present Study

The present study sought to investigate and replicate the proposed 6-factor model of the combined ICD-11 and DSM-5 trait domains using a modified version of the PID5BF+ algorithm on international PID-5 data. Additionally, we aimed to investigate the associations between the 6 trait domains and the 10 familiar DSM-5 PD in order to determine continuity between traditional PD types and the combined DSM-5/ICD-11 traits. We expected the pattern of associations to be consistent with previous research on these domains in relation to familiar PD types [20, 21].

Materials and Methods

Instruments

In the current study we employed a modified version of the PID5BF+ [19], which comprises 36 items that were used to measure 6 domains by means of 18 facets.

The original PID5BF+ is a 34-item self-report form developed from the original PID-5 item pool to delineate the combined DSM-5 and ICD-11 trait features within 6 domains (i.e., negative affectivity, detachment, antagonism, disinhibition, anankastia, and psychoticism). The selection of the 34 PID5BF+ items was done by Kerber et al. [19] using ant colony optimization algorithms, which is a computational method that has been proven to be very effective for item selection tasks. For further details about the construction of the PID5BF+ we refer to Kerber et al. [19]. This original PID5BF+ consists of 34 items which operationalize the 6 domains by means of 17 primary facets that are largely supported by meta-analytic findings in terms of high expected loadings and low unexpected loadings across the higher-order domains [13]. The PID-5BF+ operationalizes the domain of anankastia as a separate domain by the facets of rigid perfectionism (i.e., low disinhibition) and perseveration (i.e., negative affectivity), which is based on an empirically derived cross-walk between DSM-5 AMPD and ICD-11 trait domains [21, 22].

In order to further adapt the PID5BF+ to efficiently capture the primary facets represented in the ICD-11 domain of anankastia, we modified its operationalization by extracting subfacets of orderliness, rigidity, and perfectionism from the composite facet of rigid perfectionism. The extraction of these 3 anankastia facets is consistent with the initial 37-facet version of the DSM-5 trait model [12]. Accordingly, orderliness, rigidity, and perfectionism were initially distinct facets which were subsequently collapsed into 1 composite facet of rigid perfectionism due to considerable intercorrelations [12]. For the perfectionism facet, we used 2 PID-5 items that were already selected for the PID5BF+ operationalization of rigid perfectionism (item 123 and item 176). For the rigidity facet, we used the only 2 items from the PID-5 that covered this feature (item 140 and item 220). For the orderliness facet, we included 2 out of 4 possible items from the PID-5 (item 34 and item 115), which were selected based on their empirical item characteristics (i.e., item-scale correlations and internal consistency). Moreover, in this modified version of PID5BF+ we omitted perseveration (2 items) as a primary feature of anankastia because this facet was originally intended to capture features of negative affectivity as reflected by its expected loadings on the negative affectivity domain [13]. The other 30 items from the original PID5BF+ representing the 5 DSM-5 trait domains remained unchanged. The modified PID5BF+ scoring key is included in online supplementary Appendix A.

The present study used a modified PID5BF+ to operationalize the DSM-5 and ICD-11 trait domains using 3 primary facets per domain (Table 2), so that all domains are represented by an equal (and comparable) number of trait indicators. The complete modified PID5BF+ comprises 36 items, which delineate 18 facets (2 items per facet). The 6 domain scores are estimated using average scores for each domain's 3 primary facets. All of the analyzed PID-5BF+ data in the present study were derived from international samples, where the original 220-item PID-5 [12] had been administered.

We employed the Structured Clinical Interview for DSM-IV – Axis II (SCID-II) [23] as a diagnostic interview for PD in a clinical subsample (n = 142), which was derived from the Danish patient sample [see details in 24].

Samples and Procedures

In the present international collaborative study we included a total of 16 samples from different countries, regions, and populations [17, 19, 25–37]. In order to ensure heterogeneity and evade range restriction, we deliberatively incorporated diverse samples including clinical, community, student, and mixed samples. Thus, all of the data have already been analyzed, described, and published elsewhere using complete 220-item PID-5 data (see references in Table 1).

To ensure valid data, we systematically employed the PID-5 Response Inconsistency Scale (PID-5-RIS) for all samples to detect and exclude cases with random responding. The PID-5-RIS was developed by Keeley et al. [38] and subsequently validated in different studies [35, 39, 40]. We consistently excluded cases with a PID-5-RIS score of 17 or above, which is supported by the aforementioned findings. As presented and characterized in Table 1, the present study included 3 derivation samples (online suppl. Appendices 1–3) followed by 13 replication samples (online suppl. Appendices 4–13). For detailed sample and scale characteristics as well as data collection procedures for each sample, please consult the respective reference and the online supplementary material.

Statistical Approach

To test whether we could identify and replicate an empirically sound 6-factor structure of the combined ICD-11 and DSM-5 primary trait facets, we subjected a polychoric correlation matrix of the 18 facet scores of the modified PID5BF+ to an exploratory structural equation modeling analysis in Mplus 7.3 with robust

Psychopathology 2020;53:179–188
DOI: 10.1159/000507589

Table 1. Model fit indices for ESEM 6-factor structure across international samples

Appendix	Derivation samples	Reference	*n*	Clinical	χ^2 (d.f.)	RMSEA	CFI	TLI	SRMR
1	Denmark (clinical)	Bach et al. [17]	584	584	104.807 (60)*	0.036	0.982	0.955	0.017
2	Germany (mixed)	Kerber et al. [19]	1,271	684	174.549 (60)*	0.039	0.982	0.955	0.013
3	US (students)	Anderson et al. [29]	605	–	97.254 (60)*	0.032	0.986	0.964	0.015
	Replication samples (see online suppl. material)								
4	Brazil (mixed)	Lugo et al. [30]	1,281	103	119.593 (60)*	0.028	0.990	0.976	0.012
5	Czech Republic (mixed)	Riegel et al. [31]	466	125	98.277 (60)*	0.037	0.984	0.960	0.017
6	Belgium (Dutch speaking; mixed)	Bastiaens et al. [32, 33]	712	234	150.962 (60)*	0.046	0.975	0.935	0.018
7	Belgium (French speaking; community)	Roskam et al. [34]	1,529	–	118.228 (60)*	0.025	0.991	0.976	0.012
7	Switzerland (French speaking; community)	Roskam et al. [34]	494	–	83.936 (60)*	0.028	0.986	0.965	0.017
7	France (community)	Roskam et al. [34]	371	–	87.461 (60)*	0.035	0.977	0.941	0.019
8	Italy (community)	Somma et al. [35]	1,965	–	191.745 (60)*	0.033	0.985	0.961	0.013
9	Norway (students)	Thimm et al. [36]	495	–	124.425 (60)*	0.047	0.970	0.923	0.018
10	Poland (mixed)	Rowiński et al. [37]	1,088	117	149.659 (60)*	0.037	0.978	0.944	0.016
11	Portugal (community)	Pires et al. [25]	1,185	–	136.217 (60)*	0.033	0.983	0.957	0.014
12	Spain (mixed)	Gutiérrez et al. [26]	1,431	420	91.741 (60)*	0.019	0.995	0.986	0.011
13	USA (mixed)	Keeley et al. [27]	1,024	80	156,591 (60)*	0.040	0.983	0.956	0.014
13	USA (students)	Wright et al. [28]	1,826	–	284.660 (60)*	0.045	0.975	0.937	0.017

TLI, Tucker-Lewis index; SRMR, standardized root mean square residual; clinical, clinical participants; community, community-dwelling participants; mixed, both clinical and community; student, university or college students. * Significant at the 0.05 level.

maximum likelihood estimation and the default GEOMIN rotation [41]. Model fit was evaluated using the root mean square error of approximation (RMSEA), the comparative fit index (CFI), the Tucker-Lewis index, and the standardized root mean squared residual. We relied on the CFI (>0.95) and the RMSEA (<0.06) as indicators of adequate model fit [42].

Results

Derivation and Replication of the 6-Factor Structure

As presented in Table 1, model fit indices were good for the 6-factor structure across the 3 derivation samples (i.e., Denmark, Germany, and the USA) in terms of CFI above 0.95 and RMSEA below 0.06. As presented in Table 2, the 6-factor model showed expected patterns for all 6 factors in terms of loadings above 0.40. Only the facets of distractibility (Denmark) and perceptual dysregulation (USA) showed loadings slightly below 0.40.

As shown in Table 1, the 13 international replication samples also showed good model fit indices in terms of CFI above 0.95 and RMSEA below 0.06. As presented in online supplemental Appendices 4–13, each replication sample overall showed expected factorial patterns, with only few deviations that particularly applied to the facets of distractibility and irresponsibility. Accordingly, in both the Czech sample [31], the US mixed sample [27], and the US student sample [28], distractibility cross-loaded on negative affectivity and psychoticism. Likewise, in the French community sample [34], the Swiss community sample [34], the Portuguese community sample [25], and the Spanish mixed sample [26], irresponsibility primarily loaded negatively on anankastia rather than disinhibition. Moreover, in the Brazilian mixed sample [30] impulsivity cross-loaded on negative affectivity, whereas in the Swiss sample impulsivity cross-loaded on antagonism. Finally, in the Swiss sample grandiosity cross-loaded on negative affectivity.

As shown in Table 2 (and suppl. Appendices 4–13), the latent factor correlations generally indicated appropriate discriminant validity. Some differences did occur across samples in the strength and pattern of correlation coefficients among trait domains[3].

Association with Interview-Rated PD

As shown in Table 3, the associations of interview-rated PD with DSM-5 and ICD-11 trait domains were overall consistent with meta-analytic findings on the DSM-5 Sec-

[3] Associations between disinhibition and negative affectivity differed between cultures, with Spain having the strongest (i.e., 0.41) and France having the lowest (i.e., 0.20) values. Additionally, associations of psychoticism with disinhibition and psychoticism with anankastia differed between samples.

Table 2. Six-factor loading patterns for Danish, US, and German samples

	Negative affectivity			Detachment			Antagonism			Disinhibition			Anankastia			Psychoticism		
	DK	USA	GM	DK	USA	GM	DK	USA	GM	DK	USA	GM	DK	USA	GM	DK	USA	GM
Emotional lability	**0.54**	**0.62**	**0.47**	−0.09	−0.02	−0.08	−0.01	−0.06	−0.05	0.11	0.04	0.23	0.11	0.07	0.10	0.02	0.19	0.08
Anxiousness	**0.53**	**0.54**	**0.64**	0.23	0.22	0.18	−0.03	−0.04	−0.04	−0.05	0.02	0.10	0.10	0.13	0.11	0.04	0.00	−0.01
Separation insecurity	**0.48**	**0.59**	**0.69**	−0.05	−0.02	−0.01	0.04	0.13	0.04	0.20	0.13	0.07	0.00	0.02	0.00	0.07	−0.05	0.08
Withdrawal	0.03	0.04	0.02	**0.85**	**0.68**	**0.70**	−0.05	−0.03	−0.05	0.01	−0.03	0.08	0.06	0.10	0.10	0.00	0.11	0.10
Anhedonia	0.20	0.12	0.24	**0.48**	**0.59**	**0.63**	0.05	0.15	0.04	0.00	−0.03	0.11	−0.11	−0.08	−0.07	0.07	0.02	−0.01
Intimacy avoidance	−0.16	−0.15	−0.07	**0.50**	**0.46**	**0.60**	0.10	−0.04	0.02	0.06	0.23	0.06	0.04	0.08	0.05	0.08	0.05	0.08
Manipulativeness	−0.16	−0.05	−0.02	0.05	0.04	0.06	**0.60**	**0.73**	**0.77**	0.15	0.02	−0.01	0.02	0.02	−0.02	0.16	0.18	0.05
Deceitfulness	0.04	0.05	0.01	−0.04	0.02	−0.06	**0.86**	**0.68**	**0.73**	0.07	0.26	0.13	0.02	0.03	0.05	0.01	0.00	−0.01
Grandiosity	0.07	0.10	0.02	0.02	0.01	−0.02	**0.51**	**0.48**	**0.44**	0.09	−0.05	−0.01	0.07	0.15	0.10	0.12	0.09	0.26
Irresponsibility	0.04	0.03	0.02	0.03	0.22	0.06	0.17	0.20	0.23	**0.45**	**0.44**	**0.47**	−0.03	−0.10	−0.15	0.11	0.05	0.06
Impulsivity	0.03	0.03	0.11	0.01	−0.10	0.02	0.08	0.13	0.08	**0.74**	**0.55**	**0.50**	−0.02	−0.03	−0.05	−0.03	0.16	0.11
Distractibility	0.17	0.24	0.12	0.00	−0.02	0.12	−0.08	−0.07	−0.04	**0.38**	**0.47**	**0.58**	0.01	0.01	0.06	0.22	0.08	0.03
Perfectionism	0.06	0.11	0.20	0.01	0.03	0.02	0.00	0.00	0.01	0.03	0.01	−0.02	**0.78**	**0.77**	**0.66**	0.01	0.06	0.10
Rigidity	0.03	0.03	−0.02	0.08	0.06	0.06	0.05	0.13	0.02	0.01	−0.12	0.07	**0.65**	**0.72**	**0.76**	0.08	0.03	0.07
Orderliness	0.15	0.07	0.07	0.03	0.04	0.03	0.07	−0.01	0.05	−0.11	0.05	−0.08	**0.63**	**0.70**	**0.71**	0.09	0.03	0.03
Unusual beliefs	0.03	0.06	0.07	0.00	0.02	0.02	0.06	0.11	0.03	0.01	0.00	0.02	0.01	−0.02	−0.02	**0.82**	**0.75**	**0.81**
Eccentricity	0.07	−0.03	0.03	0.12	0.19	0.21	0.10	−0.05	0.09	0.15	0.22	0.15	0.14	0.06	0.13	**0.46**	**0.53**	**0.50**
Perceptual dysregulation	0.06	0.07	−0.04	0.05	−0.03	0.02	0.01	0.12	0.02	0.12	0.18	0.21	0.06	0.09	0.12	**0.43**	**0.39**	**0.49**
Latent domain correlations																		
Negative affectivity	–	–	–															
Detachment	**0.11**	**0.13**	**0.21**	–	–	–												
Antagonism	−0.02	**0.11**	0.02	0.07	**0.11**	0.03	–	–	–									
Disinhibition	**0.26**	**0.25**	**0.39**	0.06	**0.16**	**0.32**	**0.35**	**0.28**	**0.23**	–	–	–						
Anankastia	**0.27**	**0.25**	**0.24**	**0.14**	**0.16**	**0.16**	**0.13**	**0.12**	**0.08**	−0.01	−0.04	0.02	–	–	–			
Psychoticism	**0.23**	**0.20**	**0.19**	**0.20**	**0.24**	**0.24**	**0.31**	**0.29**	**0.26**	**0.35**	**0.39**	**0.36**	**0.23**	**0.18**	**0.28**	–	–	–

Danish clinical sample: $n = 584$. USA student sample: $n = 605$. German mixed sample: $n = 1,271$. Expected primary loadings are in bold. The matrix at the bottom shows latent factor correlations, where coefficients in bold are significant at the 0.05 level. DK, Denmark; GM, Germany.

Table 3. Association with interview-rated DSM-5 PD criterion counts

	Modified PID5BF+ ICD-11 and DSM-5 trait domains					
	negative affectivity	detachment	antagonism	disinhibition	anankastia	psychoticism
Paranoid	0.37	0.29	0.33	0.23	0.21	0.36
Schizoid	–0.18	0.28	0.22	0.06	0.05	0.14
Schizotypal	0.11	0.19	0.24	0.19	0.15	0.57
Antisocial	–0.36	0.00	0.53	0.33	0.03	0.20
Borderline	0.45	0.25	0.25	0.44	0.25	0.35
Histrionic	0.26	–0.04	0.36	0.36	0.22	0.21
Narcissistic	–0.11	–0.01	0.67	0.27	0.12	0.30
Avoidant	0.50	0.33	–0.11	0.09	0.21	0.03
Dependent	0.47	0.16	–0.01	0.30	0.05	0.22
Obsessive-compulsive	0.26	0.09	0.17	0.04	0.66	0.26

n = 142. All coefficients above 0.17 are significant at the 0.05 level, and coefficients above 0.21 are significant at the 0.001 level.

tion III [20] as well as research on the ICD-11 trait domains [21]. Paranoid PD was predominantly related to negative affectivity, psychoticism, antagonism, and detachment, in that order. Schizoid PD was related to Detachment and secondarily to antagonism and lack of negative affectivity. Schizotypal PD was related to psychoticism and secondarily to antagonism and detachment. Antisocial PD was related to antagonism, low negative affectivity, and disinhibition. Borderline PD was related to negative affectivity, disinhibition, and psychoticism. Histrionic PD was related to antagonism, disinhibition, and negative affectivity. Narcissistic PD was related to antagonism and secondarily to psychoticism and disinhibition. Avoidant PD was related to negative affectivity and detachment and secondarily to anankastia. Dependent PD was related to negative affectivity and disinhibition. Finally, obsessive-compulsive PD was related to anankastia and secondarily to negative affectivity and psychoticism.

In order to inspect the difference between the original PID5BF+ algorithm and the modified PID5BF+ algorithm, we compared their correlations with PD criterion counts. First, we found the modified PID5BF+ anankastia domain to be more strongly correlated with obsessive-compulsive PD (r = 0.66) relative to the original PID-5BF+ anankastia domain (r = 0.48). Moreover, the original PID5BF+ anankastia domain showed a stronger mean correlation with other PD (r_m = 0.18) relative to the modified PID5BF+ anankastia domain (r_m = 0.14). These patterns suggest that the modified PID5BF+ has better sensitivity and specificity for obsessive-compulsive PD relative to the original PID5BF+. However, both operationalizations of anankastia seem useful for the purpose of capturing features of compulsivity. In any case, when correlating the original PID5BF+ anankastia score with the modified PID5BF+ anankastia score, using the mixed German sample, we found the 2 domain scores to be substantially overlapping (r = 0.80).

Discussion

In the present study we investigated and replicated a 6-factor model of the combined ICD-11 and DSM-5 trait domains (i.e., negative affectivity, detachment, antagonism, disinhibition, anankastia, and psychoticism) across international samples using a modified version of the PID5BF+ (36 items). We also found that the 6 modified PID5BF+ domains overall showed good discriminant validity and meaningful continuity with familiar interview-rated PD, consistent with previous findings on the PID-5 [20, 21, 24]. Notably, this 6-domain structure of personality traits aligns with the 6-domain trait model originally proposed for DSM-5 [11]. In general, the 18 modified PID5BF+ facets showed expected loadings with good model fits across different countries and populations. The most evident deviating pattern applied to irresponsibility (negative cross-loading on anankastia) and distractibility (cross-loadings on negative affectivity and psychoticism), which is consistent with PID-5 research on ICD-11 traits [17] and DSM-5 traits [13], respectively. In the following sections, our findings will be further discussed in relation to the path going forward for ICD-11 and DSM-5.1.

A Feasible Facet-Level Portrait of ICD-11 Trait Qualifiers

In contrast to the more parsimonious ICD-11 trait domain model, the DSM-5 AMPD trait system allows clinicians to specify 25 trait facets. According to the ICD-11 Working Group for the Revision of Personality Disorders, such facet level information was thought to add unnecessary complexity to the classification [43, 44]. Nevertheless, reference to potential facet level features is included within the description of the five ICD-11 domains, but there is no coding for specific facets [7]. Even though ICD-11 trait qualifiers are only coded at the domain level, which seems most feasible for most WHO member countries, more specialized practitioners often desire a number of facet descriptors to guide their conceptualization and treatment planning [45]. The present study shows that primary features of each ICD-11 trait domain may be reliably and validly portrayed using specific DSM-5 trait facets, which also works across different countries and languages. In cases where practitioners or researchers would only want a profile of the 5 established ICD-11 trait domain qualifiers, the 6 items comprising the psychoticism domain may be omitted, which would yield a reduced 30-item version.

Would DSM-5 Benefit from a Separate Domain of Compulsivity/Anankastia?

The DSM-5 trait system describes features of anankastia/compulsivity in terms of a low score on disinhibition (i.e., rigid perfectionism). However, when looking at the latent factor correlations reported in Table 2 (and suppl. Appendices 4–13), there are no substantial negative correlations between disinhibition and anankastia, which somewhat speaks against using the low end of disinhibition as measure of anankastia as suggested in the DSM-5 proposal [11, 12]. This is consistent with previous research supporting a distinct and psychometrically sound domain of anankastia [17, 46]. Most importantly, it might not be straightforward or clinically meaningful for practitioners to specify a code for "low disinhibtion" or "lack of disinhibition" in order to highlight this trait feature, and lack of something does not necessarily mean presence of something else. In fact, it is not uncommon that a rather complex PD is characterized by both compulsivity and disinhibition [47], which therefore requires that these 2 features can be specified simultaneously using 2 separate codes. Also, when employed for research and screening purposes, it would not be possible to measure these 2 features at the same time if each were only represented by polar opposites within a single dimension (i.e., disinhibition vs. compulsivity dimension). Moreover, experts on compulsivity have called for a more multidimensional profile of anankastia in response to the current DSM-5 AMPD model in which compulsivity/anankastia is only represented by the facet of rigid perfectionism (low disinhibition) along with a secondary facet of perseveration (negative affectivity) [48, 49]. Thus, we suggest that a future DSM-5.1 should include a separate domain of anankastia/compulsivity just as in the original PD proposal for DSM-5 [11]. We also endorse the inclusion of multiple facets of anankastia/compulsivity (e.g., perfectionism, orderliness, and rigidity), which can be represented by 2 items per facet as demonstrated in the present study.

Issues Related to the Domain of Psychoticism and Psychotic-Like Features

In the initial DSM-5 proposal, the psychoticism domain was labelled "schizotypy" including facets of unusual perceptions, unusual beliefs, eccentricity, cognitive dysregulation, and dissociation proneness [11]. For empirical reasons, these facets were eventually collapsed into unusual beliefs and experiences, eccentricity, and cognitive and perceptual dysregulation within the higher-order domain of psychoticism [12], as operationalized in the present study. This maladaptive domain can be said to refer to a dimension[4] ranging from normal dissociative, imaginative, and unconventional features to more extreme schizophrenia-like features (e.g., "Sometimes I can influence other people just by sending my thoughts to them."). On this continuum, the DSM-5 captures features of schizotypy that are closer to the "normal" end, characterized by eccentric appearance or some cognitive disorganization [50]. Thus, the DSM-5 definition of psychoticism can be said to refer to a normal variation of schizophrenia liability including features of dissociation proneness. Importantly, this schizotypal-oriented definition of psychoticism should not be equated with the broader concept of Eysenck [51] of psychoticism characterized by features such as aggressiveness, impulsivity, and creativity, which he believed were linked to vulnerability to psychosis. In other words, the concept of Eysenck [51] of psychoticism is more related to disinhibition and antagonism, whereas his trait of creativity may be somewhat related to psychoticism or schizotypy in terms of unconventionality [52]. Nevertheless, consistent with the

[4] From the perspective of "polar opposites" the healthy end of this dimension may be conceptualized as "lucidity" [45].

Psychopathology 2020;53:179–188
DOI: 10.1159/000507589

model of Eysenck [51], the majority of PID-5 research on psychoticism has shown substantial associations between psychoticism and disinhibition [13]. Likewise, the strongest interfactor correlations in the present study applied to these 2 domains (Table 2). Finally, the DSM-5 AMPD operationalization of psychoticism partially captures features of borderline PD in terms of cognitive and perceptual dysregulation, which includes features of dissociation proneness [21, 53, 54].

In contrast to the DSM-5 approach (Sections II and III), the ICD-11 PD classification does not provide any code for schizotypy or psychoticism because such features are coded within schizophrenia and other primary psychotic disorders. However, many clinicians and researchers may stay loyal to the more familiar DSM-5 schizotypal personality features including the growing body of research, yet the ICD-11 classification of PD severity may rely on whether the patient experiences "dissociative states or psychotic-like beliefs or perceptions" and/or is "highly eccentric," which may resemble certain features of schizotypy or psychoticism. Accordingly, the ICD-11 approach is somewhat consistent with the traditional structural approach to classification of personality organization (e.g., neurotic, borderline, and psychotic levels), in which the lowest and most severe borderline levels may involve transient psychotic states [55]. In other words, the ICD-11 approach can be said to conceptualize and classify the capacity for reality testing (i.e., "accuracy of situational and interpersonal appraisals") according to level of PD severity, and not as a distinct trait domain [22].

Notably, the ICD-11 severity-related features of psychotic-like perceptions must be associated with situations of high affective arousal, which does not necessarily apply to the DSM-5 trait domain of psychoticism. For example, a person characterized by DSM-5 psychoticism may be able to live a satisfactory life with low distress despite eccentricity and somewhat odd beliefs. In contrast, a person characterized by ICD-11 severe PD with psychotic-like experiences in situations of high affective arousal may be viewed as having a highly vulnerable inner structure with strongly immature defense mechanisms when placed in unstructured situations or being under pressure [56]. Thus, the ICD-11 classification of PD severity according to "reality testing" may not simply be exchanged with the trait of psychoticism and vice versa.

We therefore propose that a future harmonization between ICD-11 and DSM-5.1 covers both the ICD-11 trait domains along with the current DSM-5 AMPD domain of psychoticism, which is consistent with the 6-domain model supported in the present study.

Towards a New PD Trait Model in DSM-5.1

It is important to underscore that the ICD-11 classification of PD is not just an "international" alternative to the American DSM-5 because, at the end of the day, the ICD-11 is the only authoritative nomenclature, even in countries such as the USA, Australia, and the UK. Thus, even the many practitioners who swear allegiance to the DSM-5 must eventually use the ICD-11 for coding purposes (e.g., national statistics, legal decisions, and health insurance). For this particular purpose, it seems reasonable that the DSM-5 framework aligns as much as possible with the ICD-11. Unless the American Psychiatric Association (APA) choses to forgo publishing another edition of the DSM and instead adopt the ICD-11 of the WHO (which could be an ideal solution),[5] we believe that a future DSM-5.1 revision might be substantially improved by further alignment with the authoritative ICD-11 in terms of including the same trait domain qualifiers, which is empirically supported in the present study across different countries and populations.

Limitations and Future Directions

The findings of the present study should be considered in the light of certain limitations and future directions. First, because the modified PID5BF+ data (36 items) used in the present study was extracted from complete 220-item PID-5 data, we suggest that future research conduct independent evaluations of the 36-item modified PID-5BF+ without using the algorithm for the complete 220-item original PID-5. Second, the present study primarily included samples from Western, educated, industrialized, rich, and democratic (WEIRD) societies, and we therefore encourage future research to include samples from non-WEIRD countries in order to further generalize the global replicability [57]. Third, it was beyond the scope of the present study to employ more stringent tests of factor congruence and measurement invariance across countries, languages, gender, age groups, and clinical status, and we therefore encourage future research to pursue this aim. Fourth, future research should investigate convergence with another measure of ICD-11 traits such as the Personality Inventory for ICD-11 (PiCD) [58]. Finally, future research should aim to establish norm values from representative samples to guide interpretation of individual PID5BF+ test scores.

[5] One official and freely accessible classification of mental disorders seems most appropriate and feasible for global mental health care, including WHO member countries that have local or independent classification systems (e.g., USA and Japan).

Acknowledgement

The present paper is dedicated to Erik Simonsen, MD, in celebration of his 70th birthday this year. Prof. Simonsen is a professor of Clinical Psychiatry at the Faculty of Health and Medical Sciences, University of Copenhagen, and founder and director of the Institute of Personality Theory and Psychopathology (IPTP) since 1989. As cofounder of the International Society for the Study of Personality Disorders (ISSPD), Prof. Simonsen spent much of his career paving the way for international dialogue within this field. More than 30 years ago, he invited prominent scholars and clinicians from around the world to the first ISSPD congress in Copenhagen, Denmark. Prof. Simonsen (in collaboration with Thomas A. Widiger) was later entrusted by the NIMH, the WHO, and the APA to take the lead in preparing the grounds for a reclassification of PD. He also founded the World Psychiatric Association (WPA) Section on Personality Disorders and chaired the WPA/ISSPD Educational Program on Personality Disorders. In the spirit of Prof. Simonsen's efforts for international dialogue and collaboration, the present work gathered contemporary PD researchers from around the world in order to establish the international validity of a feasible and empirically robust measure of PD traits that harmonizes and integrates the ICD-11 and the DSM-5 nosologies.

Statement of Ethics

This research was conducted ethically in accordance with the World Medical Association Declaration of Helsinki. Subjects have given their informed consent and ethical approval was not required due to the nature of this study.

Disclosure Statement

The authors have no conflict of interests to declare.

Author Contributions

B.B. drafted this paper and initiated data analyses in collaboration with J.Z., A.K., A.F., and A.S.; A.A., T.B., L.C., F.G., S.E.S.O., R.P., K.D.R., J.-P.R., I.R., M.S., A.S., L.S., W.S., J.C.T., J.W.K., and A.G.C.W. provided data and critically reviewed/revised this work.

References

1 Volkert J, Gablonski TC, Rabung S. Prevalence of personality disorders in the general adult population in Western countries: systematic review and meta-analysis. Br J Psychiatry. 2018 Dec;213(6):709–15.

2 Beckwith H, Moran PF, Reilly J. Personality disorder prevalence in psychiatric outpatients: a systematic literature review. Pers Ment Health. 2014 May;8(2):91–101.

3 Tyrer P, Reed GM, Crawford MJ. Classification, assessment, prevalence, and effect of personality disorder. Lancet. 2015 Feb; 385(9969):717–26.

4 Fossati A. European perspectives on personality disorders: knowing a complex history for a (hopefully) bright future. Pers Ment Health. 2011;5(2):132–43.

5 Keeley JW, Reed GM, Roberts MC, Evans SC, Medina-Mora ME, Robles R, et al. Developing a science of clinical utility in diagnostic classification systems field study strategies for ICD-11 mental and behavioral disorders. Am Psychol. 2016 Jan;71(1):3–16.

6 Zimmermann J, Kerber A, Rek K, Hopwood CJ, Krueger RF. A Brief but Comprehensive Review of Research on the Alternative DSM-5 Model for Personality Disorders. Curr Psychiatry Rep. 2019 Aug;21(9):92.

7 World Health Organization. ICD-11 clinical descriptions and diagnostic guidelines for mental and behavioural disorders. Geneva: WHO; 2019.

8 Bach B, Presnall-Shvorin J. Using DSM-5 and ICD-11 personality traits in clinical treatment. In: Gratz KL, Lejuez C, editors. Cambridge handbook of personality disorders. 1st ed. Cambridge: Cambridge University Press; 2020. p. 450–67.

9 Crego C, Widiger TA. The Conceptualization and Assessment of Schizotypal Traits: A Comparison of the FFSI and PID-5. J Pers Disord. 2017 Oct;31(5):606–23.

10 Lenzenweger MF. Schizotypy, schizotypic psychopathology and schizophrenia. World Psychiatry. 2018 Feb;17(1):25–6.

11 Skodol AE, Clark LA, Bender DS, Krueger RF, Morey LC, Verheul R, et al. Proposed changes in personality and personality disorder assessment and diagnosis for DSM-5 Part I: description and rationale. Pers Disord. 2011 Jan; 2(1):4–22.

12 Krueger RF, Derringer J, Markon KE, Watson D, Skodol AE. Initial construction of a maladaptive personality trait model and inventory for DSM-5. Psychol Med. 2012 Sep;42(9): 1879–90.

13 Watters CA, Bagby RM. A meta-analysis of the five-factor internal structure of the Personality Inventory for DSM-5. Psychol Assess. 2018 Sep;30(9):1255–60.

14 Bach B, El Abiddine FZ. Empirical structure of DSM-5 and ICD-11 personality disorder traits in Arab-speaking Algerian culture. Int J Ment Health. 2020;1–15.

15 Maples JL, Carter NT, Few LR, Crego C, Gore WL, Samuel DB, et al. Testing whether the DSM-5 personality disorder trait model can be measured with a reduced set of items: an item response theory investigation of the Personality Inventory for DSM-5. Psychol Assess. 2015 Dec;27(4): 1195–210.

16 Bach B, Maples-Keller JL, Bo S, Simonsen E. The alternative DSM-5 personality disorder traits criterion: A comparative examination of three self-report forms in a Danish population. Pers Disord. 2016 Apr;7(2):124–35.

17 Bach B, Sellbom M, Kongerslev M, Simonsen E, Krueger RF, Mulder R. Deriving ICD-11 personality disorder domains from dsm-5 traits: initial attempt to harmonize two diagnostic systems. Acta Psychiatr Scand. 2017 Jul;136(1):108–17.

18 Sellbom M, Solomon-Krakus S, Bach B, Bagby RM. Validation of Personality Inventory for DSM-5 (PID-5) algorithms to assess ICD-11 personality trait domains in a psychiatric sample. Psychol Assess. 2020 Jan;32(1):40–9.

19 Kerber A, Schultze M, Müller S, Rühling RM, Wright AG, Spitzer C, Krueger RF, et al. Development of a short and ICD-11 compatible measure for DSM-5 maladaptive personality traits using ant colony optimization algorithms.. Available from: https://doi.org/10.31234/osf.io/rsw54.

20 Watters CA, Bagby RM, Sellbom M. Meta-analysis to derive an empirically based set of personality facet criteria for the alternative DSM-5 model for personality disorders. Personal Disord. 2019 Mar;10(2):97-104.

21 Bach B, Sellbom M, Skjernov M, Simonsen E. ICD-11 and DSM-5 personality trait domains capture categorical personality disorders: finding a common ground. Aust N Z J Psychiatry. 2018 May;52(5):425–34.

22 Bach B, First MB. Application of the ICD-11 classification of personality disorders. BMC Psychiatry. 2018 Oct;18(1):351.

23 First MB, Gibbon M, Spitzer RL, Benjamin LS, Williams JB. User's guide for the structured clinical interview for DSM-IV axis II personality disorders: SCID-II. Washington: American Psychiatric Press; 1997.

24 Bach B, Anderson J, Simonsen E. Continuity between interview-rated personality disorders and self-reported DSM-5 traits in a Danish psychiatric sample. Pers Disord. 2017 Jul; 8(3):261–7.

25 Pires R, Sousa Ferreira A, Gonçalves B, Henriques-Calado J, Paulino M. The Portuguese version of the Personality Inventory for the DSM-5 in a community and a clinical sample. Pers Ment Health. 2019 Feb;13(1):40–52.

26 Gutiérrez F, Aluja A, Peri JM, Calvo N, Ferrer M, Baillés E, et al. Psychometric Properties of the Spanish PID-5 in a Clinical and a Community Sample. Assessment. 2017 Apr;24(3): 326–36.

27 Keeley JW, Flanagan EH, McCluskey DL. Functional impairment and the DSM-5 dimensional system for personality disorder. J Pers Disord. 2014 Oct;28(5):657–74.

28 Wright AG, Thomas KM, Hopwood CJ, Markon KE, Pincus AL, Krueger RF. The hierarchical structure of DSM-5 pathological personality traits. J Abnorm Psychol. 2012 Nov; 121(4):951–7.

29 Anderson JL, Sellbom M, Bagby RM, Quilty LC, Veltri CO, Markon KE, et al. On the convergence between PSY-5 domains and PID-5 domains and facets: implications for assessment of DSM-5 personality traits. Assessment. 2013 Jun;20(3):286–94.

30 Lugo V, de Oliveira SE, Hessel CR, Monteiro RT, Pasche NL, Pavan G, et al. Evaluation of DSM-5 and ICD-11 personality traits using the Personality Inventory for DSM-5 (PID-5) in a Brazilian sample of psychiatric inpatients. Pers Ment Health. 2019 Feb;13(1):24–39.

31 Riegel KD, Ksinan AJ, Samankova D, Preiss M, Harsa P, Krueger RF. Unidimensionality of the personality inventory for DSM-5 facets: evidence from two Czech-speaking samples. Pers Ment Health. 2018 Nov;12(4):281–97.

32 Bastiaens T, Claes L, Smits D, De Clercq B, De Fruyt F, Rossi G, et al. The Construct Validity of the Dutch Personality Inventory for DSM-5 Personality Disorders (PID-5) in a Clinical Sample. Assessment. 2016 Feb;23(1):42–51.

33 Bastiaens T, Smits D, De Hert M, Vanwalleghem D, Claes L. DSM-5 section III personality traits and section II personality disorders in a Flemish community sample. Psychiatry Res. 2016 Apr;238(2016):290–8.

34 Roskam I, Galdiolo S, Hansenne M, Massoudi K, Rossier J, Gicquel L, et al. The Psychometric Properties of the French Version of the Personality Inventory for DSM-5. PLoS One. 2015 Jul;10(7):e0133413.

35 Somma A, Borroni S, Kelley SE, Edens JF, Fossati A. Further evidence for the validity of a response inconsistency scale for the Personality Inventory for DSM-5 in Italian community-dwelling adolescents, community-dwelling adults, and clinical adults. Psychol Assess. 2018 Jul;30(7):929–40.

36 Thimm JC, Jordan S, Bach B. Hierarchical Structure and Cross-Cultural Measurement Invariance of the Norwegian Version of the Personality Inventory for DSM-5. J Pers Assess. 2017 Mar-Apr;99(2):204–10.

37 Rowiński T, Kowalska-Dąbrowska M, Strus WS, Cieciuch J, Czuma I, Żechowski C, et al. Measurement of pathological personality traits according to Section III of the DSM-5: A Polish adaptation of PID-5. Part II – Empirical results. Psychiatr Pol. 2018 May; 2674(1):1–16.

38 Keeley JW, Webb C, Peterson D, Roussin L, Flanagan EH. Development of a Response Inconsistency Scale for the Personality Inventory for DSM-5. J Pers Assess. 2016 Jul-Aug; 98(4):351–9.

39 Bagby RM, Sellbom M. The Validity and Clinical Utility of the Personality Inventory for DSM-5 Response Inconsistency Scale. J Pers Assess. 2018 Jul-Aug;100(4):398–405.

40 Lowmaster SE, Hartman MJ, Zimmermann J, Baldock ZC, Kurtz JE. Further validation of the Response Inconsistency Scale for the Personality Inventory for DSM-5. J Pers Assess. 2019 Oct;(Oct):1–8.

41 Muthén LK, Muthén BO. Mplus user's guide. 6th ed. Los Angeles (CA): Muthén & Muthén; 2012.

42 Hu LT, Bentler PM. Cutoff criteria for fit indexes in covariance structure analysis: conventional criteria versus new alternatives. Struct Equ Modeling. 1999;6(1):1–55.

43 Mulder RT, Newton-Howes G, Crawford MJ, Tyrer PJ. The central domains of personality pathology in psychiatric patients. J Pers Disord. 2011 Jun;25(3):364–77.

44 Tyrer P, Crawford M, Mulder RT, Blashfield R, Farnam A, Fossati A, et al. The rationale for the reclassification of personality disorder in the 11th revision of the International Classification of Diseases (ICD-11). Pers Ment Health. 2011 Nov;5(4):246–59.

45 Bach B, Markon K, Simonsen E, Krueger RF. Clinical utility of the DSM-5 alternative model of personality disorders: six cases from practice. J Psychiatr Pract. 2015 Jan;21(1):3–25.

46 Mulder RT, Horwood J, Tyrer P, Carter J, Joyce PR. Validating the proposed ICD-11 domains. Pers Ment Health. 2016 May;10(2): 84–95.

47 Chamberlain SR, Stochl J, Redden SA, Grant JE. Latent traits of impulsivity and compulsivity: toward dimensional psychiatry. Psychol Med. 2018 Apr;48(5):810–21.

48 Ayearst LE, Flett GL, Hewitt PL. Where is multidimensional perfectionism in DSM-5? A question posed to the DSM-5 personality and personality disorders work group. Pers Disord. 2012 Oct;3(4):458–69.

49 Stoeber J. Multidimensional perfectionism and the DSM-5 personality traits. Pers Individ Dif. 2014 Jul;64:115–20.

50 Rawlings D, Williams B, Haslam N, Claridge G. Taxometric analysis supports a dimensional latent structure for schizotypy. Pers Individ Dif. 2008;44(8):1640–51.

51 Eysenck HJ. The definition and measurement of psychoticism. Pers Individ Dif. 1992;13(7): 757–85.

52 Widiger TA, Simonsen E. Alternative dimensional models of personality disorder: finding a common ground. J Pers Disord. 2005 Apr; 19(2):110–30.

53 Sellbom M, Sansone RA, Songer DA, Anderson JL. Convergence between DSM-5 Section II and Section III diagnostic criteria for borderline personality disorder. Aust N Z J Psychiatry. 2014 Apr;48(4):325–32.

54 Bach B, Sellbom M. Continuity between DSM-5 Categorical Criteria and Traits Criteria for Borderline Personality Disorder. Can J Psychiatry. 2016 Aug;61(8):489–94.

55 Caligor E, Kernberg OF, Clarkin JF, Yeomans FE. Psychodynamic Therapy for Personality Pathology: Treating Self and Interpersonal Functioning. Arlington, VA, US: American Psychiatric Publishing; 2018.

56 Skodol AE, Gunderson JG, Pfohl B, Widiger TA, Livesley WJ, Siever LJ. The borderline diagnosis I: psychopathology, comorbidity, and personality structure. Biol Psychiatry. 2002 Jun;51(12):936–50.

57 Henrich J, Heine SJ, Norenzayan A. The weirdest people in the world? Behav Brain Sci. 2010 Jun;33(2-3):61–83.

58 Oltmanns JR, Widiger TA. A self-report measure for the ICD-11 dimensional trait model proposal: the personality inventory for ICD-11. Psychol Assess. 2018 Feb;30(2):154–69.

59 Maden T, Tyrer P. Dangerous and severe personality disorders: a new personality concept from the United Kingdom. J Pers Disord. 2003 Dec;17(6):489–96.

60 Wilberg T, Karterud S, Pedersen G, Urnes Ø. The impact of avoidant personality disorder on psychosocial impairment is substantial. Nord J Psychiatry. 2009;63(5):390–6.

Review Article

Psychopathology

Psychopathology 2020;53:189–197
DOI: 10.1159/000507590

Received: January 17, 2020
Accepted: March 27, 2020
Published online: May 6, 2020

Integrating Structure and Function in Conceptualizing and Assessing Pathological Traits

Aidan G.C. Wright Aleksandra Kaurin

Department of Psychology, University of Pittsburgh, Pittsburgh, PA, USA

Keywords
Personality pathology · Personality traits · Structure · Function · Contextualized processes

Abstract
The Diagnostic and Statistical Manual of Mental Disorders' (5th Edition) Alternative Model of Personality Disorders includes a dimensional trait model to describe individual differences in the manifestation of personality pathology. Empirically derived quantitative trait models of psychopathology address many of the structural problems of classical diagnostic schemes (e.g., nonbinary distributions, excessive comorbidity, and diagnostic heterogeneity). However, they are largely based on the structure of individual differences in the manifestation of psychopathology. In contrast, clinical theories of personality disorder, which are the foundation of intervention efforts, are based on the function of maladaptive behavior. This distinction is akin to the difference between morphology and physiology in the broader biological sciences. A structure-function divide in the focus of empirical and clinical work contributes to a lack of integration and difficulties with translation. Here we discuss this tension and argue for the need to bridge this divide and adopt research efforts that integrate structure and function of personality traits. Specifically, we suggest that between-person structure identifies the principal domains of functioning, but to understand dysfunction personality must be conceptualized and studied as an ensemble of contextualized dynamic processes.

Integrating Structure and Function in Conceptualizing and Assessing Pathological Traits

Personality pathology occupies a challenging position in clinical research and practice. Unlike primarily affective syndromes that are often experienced as separate from the individual (i.e., egodystonic), personality pathology refers to difficulties in the most central elements of our identities – ingrained in enduring habits of thought, feeling, behavior, and how we think of ourselves (i.e., egosyntonic). As such, personality pathology is essential to who we are as persons and, when severe, it is pervasive, persistent, and difficult to characterize and treat. It often undergirds common problems like depression and anxiety, and without careful evaluation these core functional

karger@karger.com
www.karger.com/psp

Karger

Aidan Wright
Department of Psychology, University of Pittsburgh
4119 Sennott Square, 210 S Bouquet St.
Pittsburgh, PA 15260 (USA)
aidan@pitt.edu

patterns are downplayed at best and overlooked at worst. In spite of, or perhaps because of, its fundamental and pervasive nature, modern psychiatric nosology has struggled to adequately describe and define personality pathology. For the past 40 years, official diagnostic nosologies, like the Diagnostic and Statistical Manual of Mental Disorders (DSM), have organized personality pathology using a syndrome model with (~10) discrete polythetic categories. Despite some notable successes in treatment development for and changing public perceptions of borderline personality disorder, the syndromal approach to describing, studying, and treating personality pathology has proven to have limited clinical utility and resulted in a stagnating, if not degenerating, research program.

By the time preparation of the DSM-5 [1] began, it had become apparent that by merging heterogeneous and fuzzy symptom sets with diagnostic cutoffs the model fails to faithfully represent clinical or empirical reality in a sufficiently meaningful way [2]. Thus, an effort was made to fundamentally revise the description and diagnosis of personality pathology. What ultimately came to be known as the Alternative DSM-5 Model for Personality Disorders (AMPD) sought to combine a detailed core definition of personality pathology largely adopted from clinical observation and theory, which emphasized impairments in self and interpersonal functioning (Criterion A), with a dimensional trait model established by psychometric procedures, which emphasized individual differences in how these impairments manifest (Criterion B). For a variety of reasons, some putatively scientific, some decidedly practical, and some undoubtedly political, this model was not adopted for the main section of the manual (Section 2), and instead was relegated to the Emerging Models and Measures section (Section 3) at the back of the book [3].

In this brief review, we focus on Criterion B and the value and challenges of incorporating a psychometrically derived personality trait model as part of a psychiatric diagnostic framework. There are well-established advantages of a dimensional trait model that we review below, yet despite these there has been and continues to be staunch antagonism towards this approach from some corners of the field. Our goal is not to further unmitigated argument in favor of dimensional traits, and instead, in a spirit of consilience, we offer an interpretation of what we perceive as the major opposition against such a model with a view towards proposing steps to integrate traits with longstanding clinical perspectives on personality pathology that emphasize failures in adaptive personality functioning. These include maintaining a coherent sense of self and mutually rewarding relationships, regulating affect, and selecting and pursuing goal-directed behavior.

The motivation for moving to what ultimately became the AMPD was to address the problematic features of personality disorder diagnosis in order to advance clinical practice and reinvigorate research into its etiology, maintenance, and treatment. The key pitfalls of the current (or any) discrete categorical model of personality syndromes include the scientific imprecision and clinical inutility of these categories, reflected in the high heterogeneity of those with the same diagnosis [4, 5], high covariation among diagnoses [6] with severe cases often described in terms of multiple personality disorder diagnoses, and the fact that many individuals with apparent personality pathology do not match any diagnoses' criteria, resulting in the overreliance on unspecified diagnoses [7]. Beyond these semantic issues, the current diagnostic cutoffs for number of criteria are deceptively precise[1] with respect to distinguishing between those with and without significant clinical impairments [8, 9]. The downstream effects of such a poorly calibrated diagnostic scheme include inactive or declining research programs dedicated to personality pathology and that treatment approaches have been developed for only a minority of these categories. As it stands now, the vast majority of diagnosis-based research is focused on borderline personality disorder, with little attention focused on other diagnoses.

A multidimensional trait model had long been proposed as a viable alternative because it addressed the fundamental imprecision and many associated problems of a syndrome model of personality disorder [10–12]. In basic personality science, contemporary trait models were derived empirically from the patterns of covariation in natural language descriptors of important individual differences in characteristic patterns of thinking, feeling, and behaving [13]. By extension, the same methods, when applied to clinical descriptors of maladaptive personality in the form of diagnoses, symptom counts, individual symptoms, or clinical scales result in models with a similar number of broad dimensions [14–16]. The trait model incorporated in the AMPD includes 25 lower-order scales and 5 higher-order domains. The process by which

[1] These cutoffs are often referred to as "arbitrary" but, as Peter Zachar noted in personal communication, this is probably something of a straw man argument and they are better referred to as "deceptively precise." They are not arbitrary because they are reasonably severe and most would agree that those meeting this threshold are significantly impaired. However, they are problematic in that they suggest a precise boundary that does not exist.

Psychopathology 2020;53:189–197
DOI: 10.1159/000507590

this model was derived involved identifying and generating the universe of content needed to faithfully capture personality pathology, developing individual scales for each construct, and submitting self- or clinician report versions of these scales to factor analysis [17, 18]. The DSM-5 pathological trait model has been highly generative leading up to and since its publication [19–21], and the International Classification of Disease – 11th Edition [22] has adopted a similar scheme for the definition and diagnosis of personality pathology.

Whereas the pattern of strong covariation among symptoms across diagnoses is problematic when dealing with putatively distinct categories, it is expected in a hierarchical trait model where signs, symptoms, and diagnostic constructs are undergirded by a set of shared processes. Psychometrically derived trait models establish dimensions that describe domains of personality dysfunction and therefore are understood to be continuously distributed, with little evidence for discernable discontinuities [23–26]. The continuous nature of dimensional traits more clearly conveys to researchers and practitioners that any agreed-upon cutoff is largely in the service of practical utility, but it is not intended to reflect of the state of nature. They can also better accommodate multiple cutoff points consistent with a clinical staging model. In addition to addressing the limitations of imprecision described above, this model provides other notable benefits, like linking to models of basic personality (e.g., the 5-factor model among others) [27, 28] and psychopathology writ large (e.g., the Hierarchical Taxonomy of Psychopathology; HiTOP) [29, 30]. This results in greater scientific synthesis, providing a shared understanding of normative and maladaptive functioning. It further makes the many additional findings of basic personality science clinically relevant and places maladaptive personality functioning as centrally relevant for understanding all of psychopathology.

However, shifting to a dimensional trait model has been met with skepticism and even derision by many prominent scholars) [31–33]. The concerns raised take on varied forms, but at their core they involve a sincere worry that a trait-based model will do violence to the clinical utility of personality disorder diagnoses and erase years of hard-won knowledge and painstakingly accrued gains in the treatment of severe forms of personality disorder [34]. The essence of this perspective is perhaps best summarized by Gunderson [p. 120 in 31]: "The existing types arose out of clinical observations of the recurrence of clinical problems within therapies – problems that were also recurrent elsewhere in their patient's lives … This is the same empirical base upon which most of medicine has developed classifications of most illnesses … No scientific model … can claim comparable clinical utility. The proposed architecture can claim to be more scientific, but we should not easily back away from any nosological system that is based on the recurrent behavioral patterns observed by multiple generations of clinicians on actual patients who are seeking help."

We feel it is important to note that these sentiments are not limited to the AMPD (and by extension the ICD-11) trait model and appear to generalize to more extensive revolutionary models of psychopathology writ large. As Weinberger et al. [p. 1,161 in 35] succinctly stated in reference to the NIMH Research Domain Criteria: "Do we need to replace categorical with dimensional diagnoses to make progress in psychiatry research? No."

But what is at the root of this skepticism? Why are trait models, despite their undeniable empirical superiority and potential to promote advances in clinical utility [36–40], viewed so pessimistically by some in the field? What we understand Gunderson [31] and others to be saying is that from the perspective of the consulting room, trait-based clinical formulation rings "tinny" and lacks the timbre or resonance of the clinical description of legacy constructs like borderline, histrionic, or narcissistic personality disorders, to name a few. As Zachar [8] argued, kind concepts are practically useful ways of integrating information. They are like models that represent certain important aspects of a case but not all features. When faced with the complexity of personality pathology with the demands of a busy clinical practice, it is easy to see how this form of pragmatism is useful despite the obvious difficulties it poses in empirical studies.

Ultimately, however, the advocates for quantitative dimensional models and clinically constructed practical kinds are talking past each other if not speaking different languages. Indeed, one is often talking the language of statistical procedures, and the other is talking about sitting in the room with a patient in all their challenging complexity. In a nutshell [p. 397 in 41]: "The clinician knows he (SIC) is dealing with process. He (SIC) cannot help but remain unimpressed with statistical procedures and results which are applied to observations made at comparatively isolated points in time, and which do not tell him something of what has been happening along the way."

The question then becomes: How do we translate each of these perspectives, the statistical/empirical and the clinical/pragmatic, into a lingua franca of personality pathology that both parties feel comfortable speaking?

The inherent tension in the field relates to what we will term the structural and functional divide [42, 43]. Being able to make translation across this divide, or integrating the 2 parts into a coherent whole, would be useful for resolving concerns with dimensional models of psychopathology while placing nosological models on solid empirical footing. Analogizing to biology, structure is akin to morphology, whereas function is akin to physiology. Knowing that there are distinct tissue types is useful for recognizing different organs (e.g., brain, liver, kidney, heart, and lungs), but structural models are static. What function each of those organs serves, and how they accomplish it, is rarely immediately and fully obvious from the differences in structures. With functional models we develop an understanding of what is actually happening – they are dynamic. In psychopathology nosology, structure has been the focus of empirical research, it has emphasized static relationships (e.g., individual differences), and it has thus far been descriptive in nature. In contrast, function (or dysfunction as it may be) is the focus of clinical theories, it emphasizes dynamic processes of pathogenesis and perpetuation (i.e., mechanisms), and it is ultimately explanatory in nature. Others have argued for this same basic point, framing it as integrating structural and dynamic perspectives on personality and its pathology [44–47].

To illustrate, consider pathological narcissism (or, more narrowly, narcissistic personality disorder) from each perspective. From a structural perspective, narcissism might be understood as reflecting maladaptive trait antagonism or more specifically described as elevated grandiosity and attention seeking [1]. From a functional perspective, these same pathological features might be described in terms of relationships exiting to serve self-esteem regulation and goal setting that is based on gaining approval from others. As another example, consider borderline personality disorder. From a trait-based perspective, borderline personality disorder is captured in large part by emotional lability, impulsivity, and hostility. A functional perspective might emphasize an underdeveloped sense of identity and insecure attachment that leave the individual vulnerable to dramatic shifts of mood and behavior poorly calibrated to the situation that serve to gratify overvalued goals or ward off fears of abandonment.

The trait-based approach provides a perfectly adequate description of the average behavior of an individual diagnosed with narcissistic or borderline personality disorder, but it fails to offer an explanation for how and why it occurs and what the maintenance (i.e., reinforcement) mechanisms may be. As such the trait-based model makes it difficult to know where or how to intervene and is therefore clinically uncompelling when considered in isolation. Indeed, anyone who only looks to the structural model's traits for the personality disorder syndromes in the AMPD would see a list of traits without having any idea of how or why these fit together. The trait model for each personality disorder construct presupposes some knowledge about the functional clinical concept. The trait model is informative, but it can be much more so if one also possesses an understanding of the functional clinical processes that are defining of personality pathology. Ideally both perspectives would inform each other and coevolve.

Integrating structure and function could help bridge the scientific-clinical divide, but doing so will require both conceptual and empirical work. We must not dismiss longstanding clinical observation and wisdom, and at the same time we should question and improve its organization in diagnostic nosologies. Quantitative statistical procedures can help to identify key structural elements of human behavior and provide incremental validity to functional clinical models. We see the following as guiding principles for these efforts:

Good description is necessary for good explanation.

The same structural model should organize adaptive and maladaptive functioning.

Understanding function requires studying contextually-sensitive within-person processes.

There is a difference between disorder and diagnosis.

We consider each of these principles in turn, although they are fundamentally interlocking and reciprocally informative.

First, without good description explanation is unachievable. This is a matter of construct validity. Without valid constructs there is little to be learned about underlying mechanistic processes. This is perhaps most evident in case control studies of personality disorder diagnoses. Because the diagnoses themselves are heterogeneous, and severe patients often have a good deal of additional pathology, it is unclear what is driving any differences between groups. Appreciation for and concern over this issue is what drives the need to move away from the current categorical model of personality disorder diagnosis. A quantitative empirical approach, as has been used to identify a hierarchy of personality traits, is intended to generate "good descriptions" of valid constructs that will fuel mechanistic research [48]. As descriptions, they serve to identify the domains of functioning that must be understood individually and as they interact within a person as a dynamical system over time.

same-age peers remains relatively stable throughout development. And while children as young as infants may evidence extreme scores on temperamental measures indicative of maladaptive trait function, they are not diagnosed with personality disorder before adolescence, because until adolescence, there is a limited requirement placed on children to acquire the new level of knowledge, skills, and cultural competence to successfully transition to an independent adult role [7]. Therefore, adolescence ushers in a qualitatively distinct maturational period where, in order to take on adult rights, responsibilities, and social and occupational roles, certain functions, subserved by qualitative shifts in cognitive and neural maturation, must come on line [7]. Many of these functions fall within the purview of identity, self-direction, empathy, and intimacy – in short, Criterion A – but coalesce around the development of self. In sum then, viewed through a developmental lens, Criterion B represents developmental continuity in personality pathology, while Criterion A represents developmental discontinuity. As such, Criterion A, but not Criterion B, can account for the onset of personality disorder in adolescence. To build this argument, I will begin by reviewing the developmental literature on maladaptive trait (Criterion B) development. I will then review the current knowledge base on Section II personality disorder in adolescence (in particular borderline personality disorder [BPD]), followed by a review of developmental research on concepts associated with Criterion A function: identity, self-direction, empathy, and intimacy, explaining how Criterion A concepts are interconnected to facilitate the development of self, thereby marking a qualitative shift in personality development – referred to as the "binding" of personality.

Maladaptive Trait (Criterion B) Development

Research conducted over the last 30 years on maladaptive trait development is best represented by the developmental personality-psychopathology spectrum approach [1–3, 8–12]. According to this approach, personality begins with temperamental traits already observable during infancy and toddlerhood, which make up the entirety of personality during the early years [8, 13]. Temperament describes the initial state from which personality develops and links individual differences in behavior to genetic endowment and underlying neural networks [14]. The original dimensions described by Thomas and Chess [15] on which children show variability in their reactions to the environment included activity level, approach/withdrawal, intensity threshold, adaptability, rhythmicity, mood, attention span, persistence, and distractibility. These dimensions were later refined to include the broad dimensions of effortful control, negative affectivity, and extraversion/surgency [4]. These dimensions appear to be valid cross-culturally [16] and demonstrate strong similarities to the structure of temperament in other animals [4] as well as to the Big Five personality factors of Extraversion (extraversion/surgency), Neuroticism (negative affectivity), and Conscientiousness (effortful control) [17]. Research investigating the links between these temperamental dimensions and symptoms of emotional and behavior disorders suggest that temperamental traits are explained by an underlying two-factor model of internalizing and externalizing behavior [18]. Similarly, research using personality (not temperament) measures has consistently replicated adult findings for a five-factor structure of typical [19, 20] and maladaptive trait function in childhood and adolescence [21], which are also subsumed by the two-dimensional spectra of internalizing and externalizing behavior [22].

The implication of this developmental model of personality-psychopathology spectrum is that internalizing and externalizing pathology constitute the severe (extreme) end on a dimensional continuum of temperamental/personality traits. For instance, externalizing disorders are seen as extreme variants of the trait of Disinhibition, and depression and anxiety constitute the extreme variant of the trait of Negative Affectivity [8]. Similarly, personality disorder is conceptualized from this perspective as extreme variants of basic traits, such that early individual differences in Emotional Stability, Extraversion, Imagination/Openness, Agreeableness, and Conscientiousness as represented by the five-factor model are seen to be meaningfully related to each of the DSM-based personality disorders in a largely similar way as has been demonstrated for adults and youth [10].

Two important take-home messages are derived from the developmental personality-psychopathology spectrum approach to personality. First, trait-defined personality is weaved into, or subserves, all manifestations of psychopathology [23]; and second, it suggests developmental continuity in personality development in that underlying structural features are understood within the same dimensional hierarchical framework across different age periods. Put differently, according to this model, whether one is interested in temperament in a 2-year-old, the Big Five in an 8-year-old, or maladaptive trait function in a 15- or 34-year-old, the same five-factor structure subserved by the two-dimensional internalizing/externalizing spectra explains the organization of behavior.

Section II Personality Disorder in Adolescence

Over the last 10–15 years, there has been a proliferation of research in adolescents using narrow-band measures of DSM-IV or DSM-5 Section II-defined personality disorder, in particular BPD. Although not in line with recent trends towards more dimensionally defined constructs of psychopathology [24], this research, which relies on more traditional DSM-based concepts such as BPD, was important for clinical reasons. Specifically, at the time of its inception, clinicians were (and sometimes still are) reluctant to identify and treat young people with personality challenges, resulting in these youngsters not receiving the help they needed [25]. Therefore, it was important, from a clinical standpoint, to demonstrate validity and reliability of DSM-sanctioned constructs such as BPD in adolescence so that the many evidence-based treatments that were developed for adult BPD could be evaluated for efficacy in young people, in addition to the development of preventative efforts. Reluctance in assessing and treating adolescent BPD was based on a variety of myths about personality disorder in adolescence, which have now been shown to be unsupported by the evidence as reviewed elsewhere [23, 26–28]. In short, we now know that Section II personality disorder, categorically defined, can be reliably and validly assessed in 12- to 17-year-olds. A wide variety of interview-based and self-report measures have been developed and validated. These measures show strong and similar psychometric properties in the assessment of Section II BPD in adolescents as in adults [6]. Using these measures, several studies have evaluated the prevalence of Section II BPD in adolescents and have shown that rates mirror those of adults – e.g., 3% in the United Kingdom [29] and the United States [30] and 2% in China [31]. Using narrow-band, continuously scored measures of borderline symptoms, research has demonstrated the onset of BPD to occur in adolescence [32]. Research using validated measures of Section II BPD in adolescence has also demonstrated very similar correlates, risk factors, and antecedents to studies conducted in adults [33]. Important in this regard have been consistent findings that Section II BPD is preceded by a comorbid pattern of internalizing and externalizing behavior in preadolescence, but not the other way round [34]. Moreover, when Section II BPD (as a continuous or categorical variable) is entered into hierarchical regression analyses to assess its incremental value in predicting relevant outcomes, it appears to add not only statistically, but also clinically significant predictive value to the model [35–37]. Therefore, Section II BPD appears to add unique predictive value to outcomes above and beyond that of internalizing/externalizing spectra disorders. Furthermore, in answer to concerns over Section II BPD being distinguishable from typical adolescent "storm and stress," studies have consistently shown Section II-defined BPD groups to show increased levels in a variety of maladaptive correlates (e.g., mentalizing, experiential avoidance, emotion dysregulation) compared to both psychiatric (adolescents with internalizing and externalizing disorders, but without Section II-defined BPD) and healthy controls [35, 38–40]. Finally, Section II-defined BPD appears to be as treatable in youngsters as it is in adults [6], with similar effect sizes for treating depression [41].

Taken together, this research, which has used more traditional criteria for establishing the validity of a diagnosis [42], has firmly established the diagnosis of Section II BPD in adolescence and its importance as a novel public health problem [25]. However, that Section II BPD indexes a form of psychopathology that can be reliably distinguished from the internalizing-externalizing spectra in both phenomenology and course should be interpreted against the background of the failure to substantiate a ten-factor solution explaining covariance among personality disorder symptoms. This failure has rightly led to concerns over the validity of the construct of Section II BPD [43–45]. While we have been in full agreement with these concerns, we have argued that Section II BPD (like Criterion A) may represent the common or core features shared by all personality pathology [46–49]. This argument is based on (1) the fact that, compared to other personality disorders, which were largely reduced to purely behavioral manifestations of personality pathology with the transition to DSM-IV, BPD still contains explicit criteria reflective of intrinsic maladaptive self and interpersonal function, and (2) recent empirical evidence that BPD appears to load exclusively onto a general factor of personality pathology (gPD), while other Section II personality disorders appear to represent specific factors or maladaptive trait constellations [50–52]. It remains, of course, an empirical question to what extent Section II BPD fully captures gPD and therefore Criterion A, but given the suggested overlap (at least in adults), it is possible to argue that BPD, gPD, or Criterion A represents an index of increased severity in psychopathology [48, 49, 53, 54], somewhere along the severity pathway between the internalizing-externalizing spectra and psychoticism [55, 56]. The question then becomes why Section II BPD, gPD, or Criterion A onsets only in adolescence. Indeed, I will argue that the suggested overlap between Section II BPD, gPD, and Criterion A becomes apparent only in adolescence, because adolescence is associated with a distinct period of rapid (and in some cases qualitative and therefore discontinuous) developmental changes in Criterion A function, which, as I will show, coalesce around the core concept of self function.

Developmental Research on Criterion A Function: Self Development as Nexus

Criterion A covers a vast array of constructs across self and interpersonal function. Regarding self function, Criterion A evaluates the extent to which an individual demonstrates integrated identity function (unique sense of self, stable and accurate self-esteem, and adequate self-regulation) as well as self-direction (meaningful short-term and life goals, adequate standards of behavior, and self-reflection). Regarding interpersonal function, Criterion A evaluates the extent to which an individual shows empathy or mentalizing capacity (comprehension of others, tolerance of differing perspectives, and understanding the impact of their behavior on others) as well as the capacity for intimacy (depth and duration of a meaningful connection with others, the desire and capacity for closeness, and mutuality of regard for others). Since Criterion A was only introduced in the DSM system in 2013, it will take time for research to accumulate on the developmental course of Criterion A function exactly as it is presented in the DSM-5. In addition, many conceptual and methodological issues have to be addressed in order to adequately chart the developmental course of DSM-5-based Criterion A function. For instance, measures of Criterion A seem to suggest a 4 (identity, self-direction, intimacy, empathy) × 3 (components of each construct) × 5 (levels) matrix, while the original conceptualization of Criterion A was suggested to be unidimensional [57]. While the field awaits these clarifications, it is worth delving into the rich, deep, and broad developmental literature on the typical development of the concepts that make up Criterion A. For instance, much is known about the typical development of identity, self-esteem, self-regulation, self-reflection, goal-setting, perspective-taking, comprehension of others, and the quality and duration of close relationships in children and adolescents, and as it turns out, all of these developmental processes coalesce to support the development of an integrated sense of self [58] (in this sense, a developmental perspective would argue in favor of Criterion A as unidimensional, or constituting a general and specific factor structure). While a full and detailed review of this literatures is beyond the scope of this article, I will present it here in abbreviated form to show how the onset of Section II personality disorder in adolescence can be explained with self development as nexus.

As Erikson [59] pointed out 70 years ago, one of the major tasks of adolescence is the establishment of a coherent and integrated sense of self. The establishment of a coherent and integrated sense of self is a precondition for successfully taking on independent and autonomous adult roles and responsibilities that facilitate contributions to society and procreation [7]. To achieve this, adolescents must successfully navigate the process of becoming a separate individual while remaining connected to others – most notably parental attachment figures. The normative and neurobiologically-based increase in risk-taking and exploration behaviors help facilitate the push towards independence [60], alongside significant advances in the metacognitive capacity for self-reflection that facilitates the ability to, for the first time, ask questions such as "Who am I?," "How do I want others to view me?," and "How do I fit into the larger social world?" [58]. The developmental building blocks of these capacities are of course observable from early childhood onwards. Preadolescent children are, for instance, able to compare different attributes about the self. We are also able to chart adaptive and maladaptive function in Criterion A-related concepts (e.g., delayed mentalizing ability, reduced empathy, problems in self-regulation). However, it is not until adolescence that young people are able to integrate varying abstract concepts into a coherent and organized whole. By late adolescence, they rely much less on direct social comparison with peers or feedback from others and begin to adhere to a view of themselves in terms of personal standards and moral beliefs associated with increases in self-directedness and self-esteem [61]. Therefore, while the disparate aspects of Criterion A are as readily observable in preadolescence as are traits, the coalescing of these aspects into a unidimensional severity continuum does not come together ("bind") until adolescence. Here, I argue for self as the nexus around Criterion A aspects coalesces.

McAdams and Olson [62] state that it is during adolescence that the "binding" of the personality begins, because, for the first time, metacognitive capacities are mature enough to handle the work of holding in balance different views of the self-in-relation-to-others. The development of self builds on a strong foundation of prior and continuing attachment security with parents and high-quality relationships with peers [63, 64]. In turn, an integrated sense of self facilitates the maintenance of strong interpersonal relationships within and outside the home. Strong attachments to parents and peers and interpersonal effectiveness are facilitated by the capacity for empathy or mentalizing, which shows rapid growth and expansion in adolescence – in some cases reflecting discontinuous maturational shifts. In particular, social neuroscience research suggest an anterior-to-posterior developmental shift in brain regions supporting mentalizing during adolescence. The well-validated linear age-related decline in dorsomedial prefrontal cortex responses during mentalizing tasks appears to be joined by linear and nonlinear (discontinuous) patterns of developmental change in other regions associated with simulation, which are highly sensitive to affective contributions [65]. The proliferation of the social brain in terms of perspective-taking, mentalizing, and empathy also allows for the development of social emotions such as shame and guilt, which facilitates adult moral functioning and allows the young adult to begin to regulate the self within his/her social context. With the expansion of the social brain, in conjunction with qualitative (discontinuous) shifts in sexual maturity and identity, adolescents are poised for adult intimacy, again informing the developing self in significant ways. Identity, self-direction, intimacy, and empathy are therefore intractably linked and remain interconnected through adolescence into adulthood to support the development of self [66].

In summary, developmental research suggests that Criterion A concepts (identity, self-direction, empathy, and intimacy) coalesce around the development of self, marking a discontinuous (qualitative) shift in development that enables the adolescent to take on independent adult role function, which is demanded from the environment. The concepts of developmental continuity and discontinuity are well known in developmental psychology and developmental psychopathology [67]. Maturation that is continuous does not change in structure or form, but follows a continuous course – for instance, height. In contrast, maturation that is discontinuous (e.g., the development of primary and secondary sexual characteristics) involves qualitative change. Whether maturation is continuous or discontinuous may be important for a variety of reasons; however, it seems more important to focus attention on the extent to which developmental changes, whether continuous or discontinuous, transform functioning. For instance, locomotion markedly increases a toddler's ability to explore and control their environment, and the development of language opens up new opportunities for social communication [67]. Similarly, the development of an integrated and coherent sense of self changes the adolescent's psychological situation to the degree that they are able to begin taking on adult social role function ("work and love"). Trait development (which represents a continuous change process) does not appear to have the same transforming quality, probably because it is descriptive in nature. Thus, while a developmental course for trait function has been described, the ebb and flow of trait development cannot account for the onset of Section II personality disorder in adolescence. Put differently, traits are unable to explain changes in behavior during different age periods and can therefore not account for the onset of personality disorder in adolescence. Here, I argue that personality disorder ensues when an integrated and coherent sense of self fails to develop, resulting in nonfulfilment of adult role function. Adaptive self function (which is intractably linked to adaptive interpersonal function) constitutes a developmental milestone that, if missed, impedes the binding of personality and ultimately the transformation from child to adult personality function.

Clinical Implications and Future Research Directions

While the empirical research reviewed in this paper reasonably points to the views presented here, several hypotheses remain untested. Longitudinal data that chart the developmental course of aspects of DSM-5 Criterion A in conjunction with measures of Criterion B and more traditional measures of psychopathology (e.g., Section II BPD and measures of the internalizing-externalizing spectra) can clarify the respective contributions of Criteria A and B in (1) explaining the onset of personality pathology and (2) disentangling (or confirming overlap) between Criterion A, Criterion B, and the internalizing-externalizing spectra. If it is indeed true that Criterion A accounts for the binding of personality into a unidimensional severity continuum during adolescence, then it is important that interventions explicitly scaffold this binding. Elsewhere, we have argued that interventions aimed at enhancing mentalizing capacity during adolescence are key to healthy personality development [54, 68]. These interventions focus on slowing down thinking and feeling around self and others so that an adaptive and integrated sense of self emerges that can effectively guide the important decisions adolescents take as they age into adulthood.

Disclosure Statement

The author has no conflicts of interest to declare.

Funding Sources

None.

References

1 De Clercq B, De Fruyt F, Widiger TA. Integrating a developmental perspective in dimensional models of personality disorders. Clin Psychol Rev. 2009 Mar;29(2):154–62.

2 Shiner JL, Tackett JL. Personality disorders in children and adolescents. In: Mash EJ, Barkley RA, editors. Child psychopathology. New York: Guilford Press; 2014. p. 848–96.

3 Shiner RL. The development of personality disorders: perspectives from normal personality development in childhood and adolescence. Dev Psychopathol. 2009;21(3):715–34.

4 Rothbart MK, Bates JE. Temperament. In: Damon W, Lerner R, Eisenberg N, editors. Handbook of child psychology. Vol. 3: Social, emotional, and personality development. New York: Wiley; 2006. p. 99–166.

5 Chanen AM. Borderline Personality Disorder in Young People: Are We There Yet? J Clin Psychol. 2015 Aug;71(8):778–91.

6 Sharp C, Fonagy P. Practitioner Review: borderline personality disorder in adolescence – recent conceptualization, intervention, and implications for clinical practice. J Child Psychol Psychiatry. 2015 Dec;56(12):1266–88.

7 Dahl RE, Allen NB, Wilbrecht L, Suleiman AB. Importance of investing in adolescence from a developmental science perspective. Nature. 2018 Feb;554(7693):441–50.

8 Tackett JL. Evaluating models of the personality-psychopathology relationship in children and adolescents. Clin Psychol Rev. 2006 Sep;26(5):584–99.

9 Forbes MK, Tackett JL, Markon KE, Krueger RF. Beyond comorbidity: toward a dimensional and hierarchical approach to understanding psychopathology across the life span. Dev Psychopathol. 2016 Nov;28(4pt1):971–86.

10 Tackett J, Herzhoff K, Balsis S, Cooper L. Toward a unifying perspective on personality pathology across the lifespan. In: Cichetti DC, editor. Developmental psychopathology. New York: Wiley; 2016. p. 1039–78.

11 Tackett JL, Herzhoff K, Reardon KW, De Clercq B, Sharp C. The externalizing spectrum in youth: incorporating personality pathology. J Adolesc. 2014 Jul;37(5):659–68.

12 Shiner RL. A developmental perspective on personality disorders: lessons from research on normal personality development in childhood and adolescence. J Pers Disord. 2005 Apr;19(2):202–10.

13 Shiner R, Caspi A. Personality differences in childhood and adolescence: measurement, development, and consequences. J Child Psychol Psychiatry. 2003 Jan;44(1):2–32.

14 Rothbart MK, Derryberry D. Development of individual differences in temperament [1981]. Adv Dev Psychol. 2013;1:37–86.

15 Thomas A, Chess S. Temperament and development. New York: Bruner/Mazel; 1977.

16 Ahadi SA, Rothbart MK, Ye RM. Children's temperament in the US and China: similarities and differences. Eur J Pers. 1993;7(5):359–78.

17 Rothbart MK. Temperament, development, and personality. Curr Dir Psychol Sci. 2007;16(4):207–12.

18 Ormel J, Oldehinkel AJ, Ferdinand RF, Hartman CA, De Winter AF, Veenstra R, et al. Internalizing and externalizing problems in adolescence: general and dimension-specific effects of familial loadings and preadolescent temperament traits. Psychol Med. 2005 Dec;35(12):1825–35.

19 Goldberg LR. Analyses of Digman's child-personality data: derivation of Big-Five factor scores from each of six samples. J Pers. 2001 Oct;69(5):709–43.

20 Caspi A, Roberts BW, Shiner RL. Personality development: stability and change. Annu Rev Psychol. 2005;56(1):453–84.

21 Verbeke L, De Caluwé E, De Clercq B. A five-factor model of developmental personality pathology precursors. Pers Disord. 2017 Apr;8(2):130–9.

22 De Clercq B, Decuyper M, De Caluwé E. Developmental manifestations of borderline personality pathology from and age-specific dimensional personality disorder trait framework. In: Sharp C, Tackett JL, editors. Handbook of borderline personality disorder in children and adolescents. New York: Springer; 2014. p. 81–94.

23 Sharp C, Kerr S, Chanen A. Prevention and early identification and prevention of personality pathology: an AMPD informed model of clinical staging. In: Oldham J, Skodol A, editors. The American Psychiatric Publishing Textbook of Personality Disorders. Washington: American Psychiatric Association [under review].

24 Sharp C. Current trends in BPD research as indicative of a broader sea-change in psychiatric nosology. Pers Disord. 2016 Oct;7(4):334–43.

25 Chanen A, Sharp C, Hoffman P; Global Alliance for Prevention and Early Intervention for Borderline Personality Disorder. Prevention and early intervention for borderline personality disorder: a novel public health priority. World Psychiatry. 2017 Jun;16(2):215–6.

26 Sharp C. Bridging the gap: the assessment and treatment of adolescent personality disorder in routine clinical care. Arch Dis Child. 2017 Jan;102(1):103–8.

27 Sharp C, Kalpakci A. If it looks like a duck and quacks like a duck: evaluating the validity of borderline personality disorder in adolescents. Scand J Child Adolesc Psychol Psychiatry. 2015;3(1):49–62.

28 Sharp C, Kim S. Recent advances in the developmental aspects of borderline personality disorder. Curr Psychiatry Rep. 2015 Apr;17(4):556.

29 Zanarini MC, Horwood J, Wolke D, Waylen A, Fitzmaurice G, Grant BF. Prevalence of DSM-IV borderline personality disorder in two community samples: 6,330 English 11-year-olds and 34,653 American adults. J Pers Disord. 2011 Oct;25(5):607–19.

30 Johnson JG, Cohen P, Kasen S, Skodol AE, Oldham JM. Cumulative prevalence of personality disorders between adolescence and adulthood. Acta Psychiatr Scand. 2008 Nov;118(5):410–3.

31 Leung SW, Leung F. Construct validity and prevalence rate of borderline personality disorder among Chinese adolescents. J Pers Disord. 2009 Oct;23(5):494–513.

32 Cohen P, Crawford TN, Johnson JG, Kasen S. The children in the community study of developmental course of personality disorder. J Pers Disord. 2005 Oct;19(5):466–86.

33 Stepp SD, Lazarus SA, Byrd AL. A systematic review of risk factors prospectively associated with borderline personality disorder: taking stock and moving forward. Pers Disord. 2016 Oct;7(4):316–23.

34 Bornovalova MA, Hicks BM, Iacono WG, McGue M. Longitudinal twin study of borderline personality disorder traits and substance use in adolescence: developmental change, reciprocal effects, and genetic and environmental influences. Pers Disord. 2013 Jan;4(1):23–32.

35 Penner F, McLaren V, Leavitt J, Akca OF, Sharp C. Implicit and explicit mentalizing deficits in adolescent inpatients: specificity and incremental value of borderline pathology. J Pers Disord. doi: 10.1521/pedi_2019_33_463 [Epub ahead of print].

36 Sharp C, Green KL, Yaroslavsky I, Venta A, Zanarini MC, Pettit J. The incremental validity of borderline personality disorder relative to major depressive disorder for suicidal ideation and deliberate self-harm in adolescents. J Pers Disord. 2012 Dec;26(6):927–38.

37 Chanen A, Jackson H, McCutcheon L, Germano D, Nistico H, Dudgeon P, et al. 02-08 A randomized controlled trial of psychotherapeutic early intervention for borderline personality disorder. Acta Neuropsychiatr. 2006 Dec;18(6):319.

38 Ibraheim M, Kalpakci A, Sharp C. The specificity of emotion dysregulation in adolescents with borderline personality disorder: comparison with psychiatric and healthy controls. Borderline Personal Disord Emot Dysregul. 2017 Jan;4(1):1.

39 Sharp C, Pane H, Ha C, Venta A, Patel AB, Sturek J, et al. Theory of mind and emotion regulation difficulties in adolescents with borderline traits. J Am Acad Child Adolesc Psychiatry. 2011 Jun;50(6):563–73.e1.

40 Jones J, Penner F, Schramm AT, Sharp C. Experiential avoidance in adolescents with borderline personality disorder: comparison with a non-BPD psychiatric group and healthy controls. Cogn Behav Ther. 2020 May;49(3):197–209.

41 Cristea IA, Gentili C, Cotet CD, Palomba D, Barbui C, Cuijpers P. Efficacy of Psychotherapies for Borderline Personality Disorder: A Systematic Review and Meta-analysis. JAMA Psychiatry. 2017 Apr;74(4):319–28.

42 Robins E, Guze SB. Establishment of diagnostic validity in psychiatric illness: its application to schizophrenia. Am J Psychiatry. 1970 Jan;126(7):983–7.
43 Widiger TA, Trull TJ. Plate tectonics in the classification of personality disorder: shifting to a dimensional model. Am Psychol. 2007 Feb–Mar;62(2):71–83.
44 Krueger RF, Eaton NR, Clark LA, Watson D, Markon KE, Derringer J, et al. Deriving an empirical structure of personality pathology for DSM-5. J Pers Disord. 2011 Apr;25(2):170–91.
45 Clark LA. Assessment and diagnosis of personality disorder: perennial issues and an emerging reconceptualization. Annu Rev Psychol. 2007;58(1):227–57.
46 Sharp C. Editorial: What's in a name? The importance of adolescent personality pathology for adaptive psychosocial function. J Am Acad Child Adolesc Psychiatry. doi: 10.1016/j.jaac.2019.10.007 [Epub ahead of print].
47 Sharp C. Calling for a Unified Redefinition of "Borderlineness": commentary on Gunderson et al. J Pers Disord. 2018 Apr;32(2):168–74.
48 Sharp C, Vanwoerden S, Wall K. Adolescence as a sensitive period for the development of personality disorder. Psychiatr Clin North Am. 2018 Dec;41(4):669–83.
49 Sharp C, Wall K. Personality pathology grows up: adolescence as a sensitive period. Curr Opin Psychol. 2018 Jun;21:111–6.
50 Sharp C, Wright AG, Fowler JC, Frueh BC, Allen JG, Oldham J, et al. The structure of personality pathology: both general ("g") and specific ("s") factors? J Abnorm Psychol. 2015 May;124(2):387–98.
51 Wright AG, Hopwood CJ, Skodol AE, Morey LC. Longitudinal validation of general and specific structural features of personality pathology. J Abnorm Psychol. 2016 Nov;125(8):1120–34.
52 Wright AG, Simms LJ. A metastructural model of mental disorders and pathological personality traits. Psychol Med. 2015 Aug;45(11):2309–19.
53 Clark LA, Ro E. Three-pronged assessment and diagnosis of personality disorder and its consequences: personality functioning, pathological traits, and psychosocial disability. Pers Disord. 2014 Jan;5(1):55–69.
54 Sharp C, Criterion A. Putting the person back into person(ality) disorder. In: Widiger T, editor. Oxford Handbook of Personality Disorders. Oxford: Oxford University Press [under review].
55 Kernberg O. Borderline personality organization. J Am Psychoanal Assoc. 1967 Jul;15(3):641–85.
56 Caspi A, Houts RM, Belsky DW, Goldman-Mellor SJ, Harrington H, Israel S, et al. The p factor: one general psychopathology factor in the structure of psychiatric disorders? Clin Psychol Sci. 2014 Mar;2(2):119–37.
57 Morey LC. Development and initial evaluation of a self-report form of the DSM-5 Level of Personality Functioning Scale. Psychol Assess. 2017 Oct;29(10):1302–8.
58 Rosen K. Social and emotional development: attachment relationships and the emerging self. London, UK: Macmillan Education; 2016.
59 Erikson E. Childhood in society. New York: Norton; 1950.
60 Steinberg L, Dahl R, Keating D, Kupfer DJ, Masten AS, Pine DS. The study of developmental psychopathology in adolescence: integrating affective neuroscience with the study of context. In: Cicchetti D, Cohen D, editors. Developmental psychopathology. New York: Wiley; 2006. p. 710–41.
61 Harter S. Emerging self-processes during childhood and adolescence. In: Leary MR, Tangney P, editors. Handbook of self and identity. New York: Guilford Press; 2012. p. 680–715.
62 McAdams DP, Olson BD. Personality development: continuity and change over the life course. Annu Rev Psychol. 2010;61(1):517–42.
63 Allen JP, Loeb EL. The Autonomy-Connection Challenge in Adolescent Peer Relationships. Child Dev Perspect. 2015 Jun;9(2):101–5.
64 Allen JP, Chango J, Szwedo D, Schad M, Marston E. Predictors of susceptibility to peer influence regarding substance use in adolescence. Child Dev. 2012 Jan–Feb;83(1):337–50.
65 Pfeifer JH, Blakemore SJ. Adolescent social cognitive and affective neuroscience: past, present, and future. Soc Cogn Affect Neurosci. 2012 Jan;7(1):1–10.
66 Montgomery MJ. Psychosocial intimacy and identity: from early adolescence to emerging adulthood. J Adolesc Res. 2005;20(3):346–74.
67 Rutter M, Rutter M. Developing minds: Challenge and continuity across the lifespan. London: Basic Books; 1993.
68 Sharp C, Rossouw T. Working with borderline teens. In: Bateman A, Fonagy P, editors. Handbook of mentalizing in mental health practice. 3rd ed. New York: Wiley; 2019. p. 281–300.

Review Article

Psychopathology

Psychopathology 2020;53:205–212
DOI: 10.1159/000509984

Received: January 22, 2020
Accepted: July 6, 2020
Published online: August 10, 2020

Disinhibition and Detachment in Adolescence: A Developmental Cognitive Neuroscience Perspective on the Alternative Model for Personality Disorders

Timothy A. Allen[a] Michael N. Hallquist[b]

[a]Department of Psychiatry, University of Pittsburgh, Pittsburgh, PA, USA; [b]Department of Psychology, Pennsylvania State University, University Park, PA, USA

Keywords
Personality disorder · Neuroscience · Alternative Model for Personality Disorders · Development

Abstract
Personality pathology often emerges during adolescence, but attempts to understand its neurocognitive basis have traditionally been undermined by problems associated with the categorical classification of personality disorders. In contrast, dimensional models of personality pathology, such as the Alternative Model for Personality Disorders (AMPD) in DSM-5, may provide a stronger foundation for neurobiological investigations of maladaptive individual differences in personality. As an example, we review studies of the adolescent development of reward processing and cognitive control and connect these systems to the normal personality hierarchy and to two dimensions included in the AMPD – Detachment and Disinhibition. We argue that by linking developmental changes in these systems to the AMPD, researchers will be better positioned to understand the relationship between neurocognitive development and the expression of personality pathology in adolescence and early adulthood.

Personality pathology often emerges and is most severe during adolescence [1]. In parallel, adolescence is characterized by widespread neurocognitive changes that influence reward processing, risk preferences, social behavior, and self-control [2]. Unfortunately, attempts to understand the links between personality dysfunction and brain development during adolescence have been stifled by the categorical classification of personality disorders (PDs) in the Diagnostic and Statistical Manual of Mental Disorders (DSM-5) [3]. Problems with categorical PDs are well-known, including the use of arbitrary boundaries to distinguish between normal and abnormal functioning, excessive comorbidity, and within-disorder heterogeneity [4].

The Alternative Model for Personality Disorders (AMPD), codified in Section III of DSM-5 [3], provides a dimensional alternative to the existing categorical PD nosology. Within the AMPD, PD diagnoses are made on the basis of (a) impairments in self and interpersonal functioning, and (b) ratings on 25 maladaptive personality traits, which can be arranged hierarchically to resemble pathological variants of the Big Five [5].

The merits and limitations of the AMPD have been articulated elsewhere [6–8], so we do not review them

karger@karger.com
www.karger.com/psp

Karger

Timothy A. Allen
100 North Bellefield Ave.
Room 756B
Pittsburgh, PA 15213 (USA)
allenta2@upmc.edu

here. Instead, we summarize specific findings from developmental cognitive neuroscience and examine their relevance for understanding normal personality dimensions and the AMPD. Furthermore, we argue that relative to PD categories, the AMPD provides a better foundation for interpreting and conducting neuroscientific studies of personality pathology, for several reasons. First, the AMPD removes arbitrary boundaries between normal and abnormal functioning, building on robust evidence that personality pathology reflects maladaptive variation in the same trait dimensions as normal personality [9]. Moreover, major traits in the normal personality hierarchy and the AMPD are conserved across species [10] and reflect neurobehavioral systems that have evolved to meet specific adaptive challenges [11]. Consequently, the AMPD may aid neuroscientific research by providing phenotypic targets that are more directly related to the organization of neural systems underlying normal and abnormal personality.

Another key feature of the AMPD is that it does not discourage the assessment of personality pathology symptoms in youth. By contrast, the DSM's categorical model advises against pediatric PD diagnoses except in "relatively unusual instances" [3, p. 647], even though numerous developmental studies have provided compelling evidence that personality pathology does not suddenly express itself at age 18 [12]. This language likely contributes to the underdiagnosis of PDs in youth and hinders research on developmental antecedents [13]. Personality pathology is the product of complex developmental pathways that begin early in life and influence subsequent adaptation and maladaptation [14, 15]. By advancing a trait model that has reasonable continuity over the lifespan, the AMPD can facilitate neuroscientific research examining how biological processes (e.g., puberty) interact with environmental and sociocultural factors to shape the development of personality.

Finally, consistent with a developmental psychopathology perspective, the AMPD acknowledges that healthy and disordered personality functioning are largely governed by the same processes and mechanisms [16]. As a result, research on the biological and environmental processes that drive typical development can help to uncover the origins of personality pathology, just as studies of personality pathology can yield insights into healthy adaptation.

Below, we review contemporary studies of reward processing and cognitive control in adolescence and consider their points of convergence with the personality neuroscience and personality development literatures. We then consider how maladaptive or extreme variation in typical adolescent neurocognitive development might be conceptualized within the AMPD, focusing specifically on Detachment and Disinhibition.

Neurocognitive Development in Adolescence: Reward Processing and Cognitive Control

During adolescence, youths navigate an array of new developmental tasks, from pursuing intense social and romantic relationships to exploring nascent autonomy [17]. Such experiences, coupled with neurocognitive development, contribute to an important period of plasticity in personality development [18]. For example, risk-taking increases in late adolescence, including drug and alcohol use, as well as risky sexual behavior [19]. Adolescents also become more sensitive to social evaluation [20]. For some, the changes that accompany adolescence can reveal or exacerbate existing vulnerabilities. Indeed, rates of personality pathology and other forms of psychopathology are elevated in adolescence [1, 21], as are other serious outcomes including non-suicidal self-injury and suicide attempts [22].

Although several accounts of adolescent changes in personality and behavior have been proposed, dual systems models are especially popular [23]. There are important variations in dual systems models, but all share a common emphasis on the development and relative balance of two neurocognitive systems: a socioemotional reward processing system that peaks during adolescence and a cognitive control system that strengthens gradually with age.

Adolescent Reward Sensitivity: Linking Dual Systems Accounts to Normal Personality

Within the normal personality literature, individual differences in reward sensitivity typically fall within the domain of Extraversion, which describes individuals who are enthusiastic, gregarious, assertive, and sensation-seeking. Maladaptive forms of Extraversion are included within the AMPD under the Detachment domain, which encompasses pathologically low positive emotionality (i.e., anhedonia) and introversion (i.e., intimacy, social avoidance) [24].

A key tenet of dual systems models is that reward sensitivity increases with development, reaching a peak in adolescence before declining or potentially plateauing

DOI: 10.1159/000509984

into adulthood [23]. Longitudinal research has not typically found age-related increases in Extraversion during adolescence, with several studies reporting a decline (e.g., Soto [25]). However, it is important to recall that personality traits have a hierarchical structure, such that broader traits account for patterns of covariation among more specific traits. Specific facets of Extraversion show divergent developmental trajectories [26], such that those most closely related to dopaminergic functioning, including sensation-seeking and social dominance, actually increase during the adolescent years [27–29].

Findings from fMRI studies typically support the dual systems perspective. For example, ventral striatum activation during reward processing peaks in adolescence and is positively associated with risk-taking behavior [30, 31]. Likewise, a broader valuation network encompassing the ventral striatum, ventromedial prefrontal cortex, and medial prefrontal cortex is more responsive to reward receipt among late adolescents than children or adults [32].

Reward-related striatal activation partly reflects dopaminergic inputs from the midbrain ventral tegmental area (VTA) [33, 34]. In animal studies, mesolimbic dopamine activity increases following unpredicted rewards and decreases following unpredicted omissions of reward [35, 36]. This pattern of activity has been called a reward prediction error (RPE) signal, which helps one to learn the subjective value of different stimuli and choose behavioral responses accordingly [37]. In humans, striatal RPEs elicited during a reward task peak during adolescence [38], though not all studies find this, potentially due to task differences or sample size [39]. Pre-adolescent and adolescent participants also show heightened functional coupling between the VTA and ventral striatum within incentivized contexts. This coupling declines with age as a function of decreasing cue-related activation of the orbitofrontal cortex [40], a region that encodes reward value and stimulates dopaminergic transmission via direct inputs to the VTA [41]. Taken together, this evidence points to a temporary increase in dopaminergic neurotransmission during adolescence, which may contribute to enhanced reward sensitivity.

Inputs from other cortical and subcortical areas to the striatum are also involved in modulating adolescent reward sensitivity. A recent meta-analysis of reward processing found that relative to adults, adolescents show greater activation in the ventral and dorsal striatum, as well as functionally connected regions, including the insula, amygdala, orbitofrontal cortex, and the anterior cingulate cortex (ACC) [31]. Developmental changes in the connectivity between these regions and the striatum appear to mirror changes in reward sensitivity. For example, connectivity between the ventral striatum and ventromedial prefrontal cortex declines with age and mediates developmental reductions in pleasure ratings following reward [42]. Likewise, the structural integrity of limbic inputs to the striatum declines during the transition to adulthood, coinciding with age-related reductions in the enhancement of cognitive performance by rewards [43].

Neurobiological research on Extraversion mostly converges with the dual systems literature. Specifically, Extraversion moderates the efficacy of pharmacological manipulations of the dopamine system, is associated with heightened activity in the ventral striatum during reward anticipation, and has been linked to increased functional connectivity between the dopaminergic midbrain and striatum [26, 44]. Furthermore, increases in the volume and activity of the ventral striatum are prospectively associated with increases in Extraversion during adolescence [28, 45]. Finally, several studies have shown that Extraversion is associated with the reward-related positivity, an event-related potential that spikes following feedback about an outcome and likely encodes an RPE produced by midbrain dopaminergic inputs to the striatum and ACC [46, 47]. Interestingly, the amplitude of the reward-related positivity increases in response to gains, but not losses, as children transition into adolescence, consistent with the prediction of dual systems models [48].

Maturation of Inhibitory Control and Concomitant Increases in Conscientiousness

Cognitive control involves the capacity to guide one's behavior flexibly and voluntarily, which requires both working memory and inhibitory control (or the ability to suppress disruptive impulses) [49]. Within the personality literature, cognitive control is closely related to Conscientiousness, a trait that describes those who are persistent, planful, and orderly[1]. Much like cognitive control, Conscientiousness has been hypothesized to facilitate the pursuit of long-term goals and promote rule-based behavior, both of which rely on the ability to avoid distractions and suppress disruptive impulses [50]. Maladap-

[1] Working memory components of cognitive control are more closely related to a facet of Openness to Experience known as Intellect [85]. However, we focus primarily on links between Conscientiousness and cognitive control here, because the AMPD does not consider intellectual functioning, and thus working memory, to fall within the domain of personality pathology.

tively low Conscientiousness is represented within the Disinhibition domain of the AMPD [51]. Disinhibition has been linked to variability in both behavioral and neurophysiological measures of error processing and inhibitory control [52]. For example, Disinhibition is associated with a reduction in the amplitude of the P3 event-related potential, a positive-going waveform that occurs following presentation of a salient stimulus in cognitive control tasks. Interestingly, P3 indices can be combined with behavioral performance measures and self-report ratings to model a cross-modal, latent Disinhibition factor [53].

From a dual systems perspective, adolescent risk-taking is conceptualized as a developmental imbalance in which the influence of the reward system outweighs a slower-developing cognitive control system. Behavioral studies have found that while many aspects of cognitive control are present early in life, they improve gradually over the course of development, remaining more variable in adolescence than in adulthood [54]. This mirrors the developmental trajectory of Conscientiousness, which tends to increase substantially in adolescence before rising more slowly through adulthood (though, it may also dip early in adolescence) [55]. Development of cognitive control depends on functional changes in the activity and connectivity of distributed regions, including dorsolateral prefrontal cortex (DLPFC), posterior parietal cortex, insula, and ACC [56]. For example, children engage the DLPFC more during inhibitory control tasks, with activation steadily declining into adulthood and mirroring performance improvements [57, 58]. Interestingly, deactivating the DLPFC using transcranial magnetic stimulation leads to increased risk-taking on a gambling task [59], whereas activating DLPFC using electrical stimulation has the opposite effect [60]. Focal damage to the area has also been linked to lower self-reported Conscientiousness [61].

The dorsal ACC is another key region in the development of cognitive control. It tends to be more heavily recruited with age, particularly in response to errors during inhibitory control tasks [57, 58]. Age-related increases in dorsal ACC activation may reflect developmental improvements in one's ability to effortfully attend to current task demands and adjust behavior accordingly as those demands change (perhaps via the recruitment of other control regions such as DLPFC) [62]. Conscientiousness is positively associated with dorsal ACC activation during inhibitory control tasks [63]. Likewise, Disinhibition has been linked to a reduced amplitude of the error-related negativity on go/no-go tasks; the error-related negativity is an event-related potential involved in error processing that has been localized to the ACC [64]. Changes in Conscientiousness also mediate the relationship between cortical thinning of the dorsal ACC during adolescence and measures of depression, anxiety, aggression, and risk-taking, consistent with the idea that poor inhibitory control is a transdiagnostic risk factor [65].

Changes in cognitive control over the course of development are tightly linked to changes in a set of highly overlapping functional brain networks – including the salience network (SN), cingulo-opercular network, and Rothbart and Posner's executive attention network [66] – all of which include the ACC and DLPFC. The basic architecture of these networks is in place early in development, but between-network connectivity strengthens throughout development, supporting improvements in cognitive control [67]. Consistent with this, network analyses show that prefrontal cognitive control regions break off into a distinct module from subcortical regions (including those involved in reward sensitivity) in individuals low in Conscientiousness [68]. The SN, whose central nodes include the dorsal ACC and anterior insula, has been linked to the detection of behaviorally relevant stimuli and the initiation of cognitive control [69]. Previous studies have shown that developmental increases in SN recruitment during inhibitory control tasks mediate age-related performance improvements [32]. Conscientiousness has been hypothesized to be related to functionally overlapping components of the salience and ventral attention networks [44], which Rueter and colleagues [70] collectively refer to as the "goal priority network." In a recent resting-state fMRI study, these authors found that Conscientiousness was associated with greater connectivity within part of the goal priority network that included the DLPFC, anterior insula, and dorsal ACC. Conscientiousness was also associated with greater coupling of these regions with functionally distinct subnetworks [70].

Disinhibition is also negatively associated with functional connectivity between the insula and DLPFC during inhibitory control [71], which suggests that the coordination of control-related regions may be critical to suppressing impulsive responses. Interestingly, cortical thickness of the insula is negatively correlated with both age and Conscientiousness, consistent with the idea that greater synaptic plasticity in the insula facilitates improved deliberation with age [72]. Conscientiousness may also be supported by better structural connectivity of the insula with limbic and prefrontal regions. For example, Lewis and colleagues [73] found that Conscientiousness was positively associated with higher fractional anisotropy (a measure of structural connectivity) in the left uncinate fasciculus, a white matter tract that connects the insula, orbitofrontal cortex, anterior temporal cortex, and amygdala. Taken together, empirical studies consistently find that the cognitive control system develops gradually with age, is related to widespread changes in control-related brain circuits, and may be a key source of individual differences in Conscientiousness and Disinhibition. Thus, heterogeneity in the development of cognitive control and reward processing neurobehavioral systems likely contributes to normative age-related risk-taking. At the extremes, variation in the development of these systems may underlie more problematic impulsive behaviors that are typically observed in personality pathology.

Linking Adolescent Neurocognitive Development to Dimensional Personality Pathology

Thus far, we have reviewed evidence supporting a dual systems account of adolescent neurocognitive development and have related individual differences in these circuits to normative personality traits, namely Extraversion and Conscientiousness. To date, however, very few studies have explicitly linked the emergence of personality pathology with prevailing accounts of neurocognitive development. By removing the boundary between normal and abnormal functioning, the AMPD provides a useful foundation from which researchers can develop and test such accounts.

How might the AMPD capture maladaptive development of the reward processing and cognitive control systems? At least with respect to reward processing, this is a complicated question. The normal personality literature distinguishes between two interrelated facets of Extraversion: an affiliative component reflecting hedonic reward consumption (also known as "liking") and an agentic component that is more closely related to incentive motivation (also known as "wanting") [34, 44]. Recent evidence has shown that the Detachment domain of the AMPD is a slightly stronger marker of affiliative Extraversion (reversed) than agentic Extraversion [74], pointing to a potential gap in coverage that may require further consideration as the system is revised over time. On the other hand, there may also be substantive reasons for this gap. While some components of agentic Extraversion are robustly linked to risk for psychopathology, others show minimal associations [75]. Sensation-seeking is a lower-order personality trait that equally blends Conscientiousness and agentic Extraversion, and it is robustly associated with externalizing problems [75]. This suggests incentive motivation may be more problematic when accompanied by at least some difficulties with top-down inhibitory control [76].

Interestingly, sensation-seeking exhibits a U-shaped developmental trajectory, peaking in adolescence in much the same way as ventral striatal activity on reward processing tasks [29]. Deviations from the typical U-shaped reward processing trajectory may be associated with the onset of externalizing problems in adolescence. For instance, one study found that smaller ventral striatum volumes in mid-adolescence predicted an increased likelihood of initiating substance use in a 2-year follow-up period [77]. In the same study, increases in reward sensitivity were associated with a greater likelihood of substance use initiation and with more self-reported alcohol use during the follow-up period [77].

Disruptions in reward circuitry during adolescence may also affect a host of other problematic behaviors that are more indirectly related to reward-seeking. For instance, activity in the ventral striatum following provocation predicts the magnitude of one's subsequent retaliation, suggesting that social status behaviors partly depend on reward-related circuitry [78]. Consistent with this, larger striatal volume in early adolescence is positively associated with aggression [79], potentially reflecting a disruption in the typical development of circuits that mediate reward-related aggression. Overall, these findings highlight the need for longitudinal cognitive neuroscience studies to address questions about the developmental trajectory of personality pathology in youth. For instance, do some adolescents exhibit time-limited personality pathology that remits once cognitive control systems exert a greater influence on behavior, while reward processing systems either plateau or decline? Does more persistent sensitivity of reward circuits predict maladaptive expressions of Extraversion in other youths? These are questions that can only be answered via longitudinal studies, preferably in high-risk developmental samples that capture the full range of maladaptive trait dimensions.

Contextualizing maladaptive cognitive control within the AMPD is more straightforward, as Disinhibition is closely related to both neural and behavioral indices of inhibitory control [53]. One AMPD facet particularly relevant to dual systems accounts is risk-taking, which was originally assigned to the Disinhibition domain but has a nearly equal negative cross-loading on Detachment (suggesting it may be the AMPD equivalent to sensation-seeking) [80]. Youths high on risk-taking may struggle to balance the lure of immediately rewarding opportunities (e.g., going to a party, having sex, trying drugs) in adolescence with the sustained effort required to attain longer-term goals, including academic and occupational achievement, stable familial and romantic relationships, and maintaining a healthy lifestyle. Given its pattern of cross-loadings, personality neuroscience researchers should consider how risk-taking depends on circuits related to both reward and cognitive control. For instance, connectivity between the dorsal striatum and inferior frontal gyrus (which is part of the goal priority network linked to Conscientiousness) is associated with an improved capacity to suppress approach responses to appetitive cues in teens and adults compared to children; only in adolescents, however, this frontostriatal coupling is also accompanied by greater ventral striatal activity [81]. This might suggest that risk-taking in adolescence reflects a biasing of cognitive control circuits related to Conscientiousness by reward signals that are encoded in the ventral striatum and more closely linked to Extraversion.

Of course, other circuits and traits that we did not cover here undoubtedly play a role in how adolescents navigate developmental challenges. For instance, another AMPD trait, Antagonism, has been linked to components of the default mode network implicated in mentalizing abilities [82] and may contribute to a devaluing of stable relationships during adolescence, in favor of short-term rewards (e.g., being more willing to manipulate or exploit a partner for immediate gain). In contrast, high scores on the AMPD's Negative Affect, coupled with risk-taking, could promote coping strategies meant to gain immediate relief from distress (e.g., self-harm, suicide attempts). The role of these traits in the development of personality pathology likely depends on the plasticity of functionally distinct networks during adolescence. For instance, networks supporting mentalizing abilities and social cognition continue to develop during adolescence [20], and extreme variations in those systems may play an important role in more interpersonal forms of personality pathology (e.g., rejection sensitivity, suspiciousness, or manipulativeness).

Conclusions

The dissemination of the AMPD and the broader shift toward dimensional conceptualizations of psychopathology in recent years are promising developments for researchers interested in the neurocognitive basis of personality pathology. By removing an arbitrary normal/abnormal boundary and reframing personality pathology in terms of empirically derived traits, the AMPD helps to build a bridge between developmental studies of neurobehavioral systems and dimensional studies of traits. Recent evidence suggests that the AMPD has clinical utility, improving communication between patients, caregivers, and providers, easing diagnostic assessment for clinicians, and helping to guide clinical decision-making [83, 84]. Integrating developmental neuroscientific evidence into the AMPD can facilitate new insights into the mechanisms that fuel personality pathology and potentially lead to innovations in assessment and intervention. Here, we reviewed how two traits in the AMPD, Detachment and Disinhibition, can be used to connect the emergence of adolescent personality pathology with the development of reward and cognitive control systems. Moving forward, we hope that this kind of integration can be used to highlight areas in the AMPD that are in need for further elaboration and refinement. Incorporating evidence from multiple levels of analysis should improve the rigor and comprehensiveness of the AMPD, making it a more clinically useful nosology.

Acknowledgement

This work was funded by the National Institutes of Health (Grant No. R01-MH119399 and Grant No. R01-MH048463 [to M.N.H.], and Grant No. T32-MH016804 [to T.A.A.]). The funding agency had no role in the preparation, review, or approval of the manuscript or the decision to submit the manuscript for publication.

Statement of Ethics

This article was prepared in compliance with internationally accepted standards for research practice and reporting.

Conflict of Interest Statement

The authors have no conflicts to disclose.

Author Contributions

Both authors reviewed and approved the final version of this work. T.A.A. was primarily responsible for drafting the manuscript. M.N.H. contributed additional writing and revisions.

References

1 Johnson JG, Cohen P, Kasen S, Skodol AE, Hamagami F, Brook JS. Age-related change in personality disorder trait levels between early adolescence and adulthood: a community-based longitudinal investigation. Acta Psychiatr Scand. 2000 Oct;102(4):265–75.
2 Spear LP. Adolescent neurodevelopment. J Adolesc Health. 2013 Feb;52(2 Suppl 2):S7–13.
3 American Psychiatric Association. Diagnostic and statistical manual of mental disorders. 5th ed. Washington (DC), 2013. https://doi.org/10.1176/appi.books.9780890425596.
4 Clark LA. Assessment and diagnosis of personality disorder: perennial issues and an emerging reconceptualization. Annu Rev Psychol. 2007;58(1):227–57.
5 Krueger RF, Derringer J, Markon KE, Watson D, Skodol AE. Initial construction of a maladaptive personality trait model and inventory for DSM-5. Psychol Med. 2012 Sep;42(9):1879–90.
6 Krueger RF, Hopwood CJ, Wright A, Markon KE. DSM-5 and the path toward empirically based and clinically useful conceptualization of personality and psychopathology. Clin Psychol Sci Pract. 2014;21(3):245–61.
7 Gunderson JG. Commentary on "Personality traits and the classification of mental disorders: toward a more complete integration in DSM-5 and an empirical model of psychopathology". Pers Disord. 2010 Apr;1(2):119–22.
8 Hopwood CJ. Interpersonal dynamics in personality and personality disorders. Eur J Pers. 2018 Sep;32(5):499–524.
9 Kotov R, Krueger RF, Watson D, Achenbach TM, Althoff RR, Bagby RM, et al. The Hierarchical Taxonomy of Psychopathology (HiTOP): A dimensional alternative to traditional nosologies. J Abnorm Psychol. 2017 May;126(4):454–77.
10 Freeman HD, Gosling SD. Personality in nonhuman primates: a review and evaluation of past research. Am J Primatol. 2010 Aug;72(8):653–71.
11 Depue RA, Lenzenweger MF. Toward a developmental psychopathology of personality disturbances: A neurobehavioral dimensional model. In: Cicchetti D, Cohen DJ, editors. Developmental neuroscience. Developmental psychopathology. Volume 2. 2nd ed. Hoboken (NJ): Wiley; 2015. pp. 762–96.
12 Kaess M, Brunner R, Chanen A. Borderline personality disorder in adolescence. Pediatrics. 2014 Oct;134(4):782–93.
13 Conway CC, Tackett JL, Skodol AE. Are personality disorders assessed in young people? Am J Psychiatry. 2017 Oct;174(10):1000–1.
14 Cicchetti D, Crick NR. Precursors and diverse pathways to personality disorder in children and adolescents. Dev Psychopathol. 2009;21(3):683–5.
15 Shiner RL, Allen TA (Livesley J, Larstone R, editors). Handbook of Personality Disorders. Developmental psychopathology. 2nd ed. New York (NY): Guilford Press; 2018. pp. 309–23.
16 Sroufe LA. Considering normal and abnormal together: the essence of developmental psychopathology. Dev Psychopathol. 1990;2(4):335–47.
17 Cicchetti D, Rogosch FA. A developmental psychopathology perspective on adolescence. J Consult Clin Psychol. 2002 Feb;70(1):6–20.
18 Soto CJ, John OP, Gosling SD, Potter J. Age differences in personality traits from 10 to 65: big Five domains and facets in a large cross-sectional sample. J Pers Soc Psychol. 2011 Feb;100(2):330–48.
19 Eaton DK, Kann L, Kinchen S, Shanklin S, Flint KH, Hawkins J, et al. Youth risk behavior surveillance. United States; 2012.
20 Somerville LH. Special issue on the teenage brain: sensitivity to social evaluation. Curr Dir Psychol Sci. 2013 Apr;22(2):121–7.
21 Merikangas KR, He JP, Burstein M, Swanson SA, Avenevoli S, Cui L, et al. Lifetime prevalence of mental disorders in U.S. adolescents: results from the National Comorbidity Survey Replication – Adolescent Supplement (NCS-A). J Am Acad Child Adolesc Psychiatry. 2010;49(10):980–9.
22 Mercado MC, Holland K, Leemis RW, Stone DM, Wang J. Trends in emergency department visits for nonfatal self-inflicted injuries among youth aged 10 to 24 years in the United States, 2001–2015. JAMA. 2017 Nov;318(19):1931–3.
23 Shulman EP, Smith AR, Silva K, Icenogle G, Duell N, Chein J, et al. The dual systems model: Review, reappraisal, and reaffirmation. Dev Cogn Neurosci. 2016 Feb;17:103–17.
24 Gore WL, Widiger TA. The DSM-5 dimensional trait model and five-factor models of general personality. J Abnorm Psychol. 2013 Aug;122(3):816–21.
25 Soto CJ. The little six personality dimensions from early childhood to early adulthood: mean-level age and gender differences in parents' reports. J Pers. 2016 Aug;84(4):409–22.
26 DeYoung CG, Allen TA. Personality neuroscience: A developmental perspective. In: McAdams DP, Shiner RL, Tackett JL, editors. Handbook of Personality Development. New York: Guilford Press; 2019. pp. 79–105.
27 Roberts BW, Walton KE, Viechtbauer W. Patterns of mean-level change in personality traits across the life course: a meta-analysis of longitudinal studies. Psychol Bull. 2006 Jan;132(1):1–25.
28 Urošević S, Collins P, Muetzel R, Lim K, Luciana M. Longitudinal changes in behavioral approach system sensitivity and brain structures involved in reward processing during adolescence. Dev Psychol. 2012 Sep;48(5):1488–500.
29 Steinberg L, Icenogle G, Shulman EP, Breiner K, Chein J, Bacchini D, et al. Around the world, adolescence is a time of heightened sensation seeking and immature self-regulation. Dev Sci. 2018 Mar;21(2):1–14.
30 Galvan A, Hare T, Voss H, Glover G, Casey BJ. Risk-taking and the adolescent brain: who is at risk? Dev Sci. 2007 Mar;10(2):F8–14.
31 Silverman MH, Jedd K, Luciana M. Neural networks involved in adolescent reward processing: an activation likelihood estimation meta-analysis of functional neuroimaging studies. Neuroimage. 2015 Nov;122:427–39.
32 Hallquist MN, Geier CF, Luna B. Incentives facilitate developmental improvement in inhibitory control by modulating control-related networks. Neuroimage. 2018 May;172(172):369–80.
33 Luciana M, Collins PF. Incentive motivation, cognitive control, and the adolescent brain: is it time for a paradigm shift? Child Dev Perspect. 2012 Dec;6(4):392–9.
34 Depue RA, Collins PF. Neurobiology of the structure of personality: dopamine, facilitation of incentive motivation, and extraversion. Behav Brain Sci. 1999 Jun;22(3):491–517.
35 Bromberg-Martin ES, Matsumoto M, Hikosaka O. Dopamine in motivational control: rewarding, aversive, and alerting. Neuron. 2010 Dec;68(5):815–34.
36 Schultz W. Behavioral dopamine signals. Trends Neurosci. 2007 May;30(5):203–10.
37 Glimcher PW. Understanding dopamine and reinforcement learning: the dopamine reward prediction error hypothesis. Proc Natl Acad Sci USA. 2011 Sep;108 Suppl 3:15647–54.
38 Cohen JR, Asarnow RF, Sabb FW, Bilder RM, Bookheimer SY, Knowlton BJ, et al. A unique adolescent response to reward prediction errors. Nat Neurosci. 2010 Jun;13(6):669–71.
39 Nussenbaum K, Hartley CA. Reinforcement learning across development: what insights can we draw from a decade of research? Dev Cogn Neurosci. 2019 Dec;40:100733.
40 Murty VP, Shah H, Montez D, Foran W, Calabro F, Luna B. Age-related trajectories of functional coupling between the VTA and nucleus accumbens depend on motivational state. J Neurosci. 2018 Aug;38(34):7420–7.
41 Sesack SR, Pickel VM. Prefrontal cortical efferents in the rat synapse on unlabeled neuronal targets of catecholamine terminals in the nucleus accumbens septi and on dopamine neurons in the ventral tegmental area. J Comp Neurol. 1992 Jun;320(2):145–60.
42 van Duijvenvoorde AC, Achterberg M, Braams BR, Peters S, Crone EA. Testing a dual-systems model of adolescent brain development using resting-state connectivity analyses. Neuroimage. 2016 Jan;124 Pt A:409–20.

43 Larsen B, Verstynen TD, Yeh FC, Luna B. Developmental changes in the integration of affective and cognitive corticostriatal pathways are associated with reward-driven behavior. Cereb Cortex. 2018 Aug;28(8):2834–45.
44 Allen TA, DeYoung CG. Personality neuroscience and the five factor model. In: Widiger TA, editor. The Oxford Handbook of the Five Factor Model. New York. Oxford; 2017. pp. 1–63.
45 Braams BR, van Duijvenvoorde AC, Peper JS, Crone EA. Longitudinal changes in adolescent risk-taking: a comprehensive study of neural responses to rewards, pubertal development, and risk-taking behavior. J Neurosci. 2015 May;35(18):7226–38.
46 Kujawa A, Proudfit GH, Kessel EM, Dyson M, Olino T, Klein DN. Neural reactivity to monetary rewards and losses in childhood: longitudinal and concurrent associations with observed and self-reported positive emotionality. Biol Psychol. 2015 Jan;104:41–7.
47 Bress JN, Hajcak G. Self-report and behavioral measures of reward sensitivity predict the feedback negativity. Psychophysiology. 2013 Jul;50(7):610–6.
48 Burani K, Mulligan EM, Klawohn J, Luking KR, Nelson BD, Hajcak G. Longitudinal increases in reward-related neural activity in early adolescence: evidence from event-related potentials (ERPs). Dev Cogn Neurosci. 2019 Apr;36:100620.
49 Luna B, Padmanabhan A, O'Hearn K. What has fMRI told us about the development of cognitive control through adolescence? Brain Cogn. 2010 Feb;72(1):101–13.
50 DeYoung CG. Cybernetic big five theory. J Res Pers. 2015;56:33–58.
51 Suzuki T, Griffin SA, Samuel DB. Capturing the DSM-5 alternative personality disorder model traits in the five-factor model's nomological net. J Pers. 2017 Apr;85(2):220–31.
52 Ribes-Guardiola P, Poy R, Patrick CJ, Moltó J. Electrocortical measures of performance monitoring from go/no-go and flanker tasks: differential relations with trait dimensions of the triarchic model of psychopathy. Psychophysiology. 2020 Jun;57(6):e13573.
53 Venables NC, Foell J, Yancey JR, Kane MJ, Engle RW, Patrick CJ. Quantifying inhibitory control as externalizing proneness: A cross-domain model. Clin Psychol Sci. 2018 Jul; 6(4):561–80.
54 Luna B, Garver KE, Urban TA, Lazar NA, Sweeney JA. Maturation of cognitive processes from late childhood to adulthood. Child Dev. 2004 Sep-Oct;75(5):1357–72.
55 Soto CJ, Tackett JL. Personality traits in childhood and adolescence: Structure, development, and outcomes. Curr Dir Psychol Sci. 2016;76(4):358–62.
56 Luna B, Marek S, Larsen B, Tervo-Clemmens B, Chahal R. An integrative model of the maturation of cognitive control. Annu Rev Neurosci. 2015 Jul;38(1):151–70.
57 Velanova K, Wheeler ME, Luna B. Maturational changes in anterior cingulate and frontoparietal recruitment support the development of error processing and inhibitory control. Cereb Cortex. 2008 Nov;18(11):2505–22.
58 Ordaz SJ, Foran W, Velanova K, Luna B. Longitudinal growth curves of brain function underlying inhibitory control through adolescence. J Neurosci. 2013 Nov;33(46):18109–24.
59 Knoch D, Gianotti LR, Pascual-Leone A, Treyer V, Regard M, Hohmann M, et al. Disruption of right prefrontal cortex by low-frequency repetitive transcranial magnetic stimulation induces risk-taking behavior. J Neurosci. 2006 Jun;26(24):6469–72.
60 Fecteau S, Knoch D, Fregni F, Sultani N, Boggio P, Pascual-Leone A. Diminishing risk-taking behavior by modulating activity in the prefrontal cortex: a direct current stimulation study. J Neurosci. 2007 Nov;27(46):12500–5.
61 Forbes CE, Poore JC, Krueger F, Barbey AK, Solomon J, Grafman J. The role of executive function and the dorsolateral prefrontal cortex in the expression of neuroticism and conscientiousness. Soc Neurosci. 2014;9(2):139–51.
62 Sadaghiani S, D'Esposito M. Functional characterization of the cingulo-opercular network in the maintenance of tonic alertness. Cereb Cortex. 2015 Sep;25(9):2763–73.
63 Brown SM, Manuck SB, Flory JD, Hariri AR. Neural basis of individual differences in impulsivity: contributions of corticolimbic circuits for behavioral arousal and control. Emotion. 2006 May;6(2):239–45.
64 Hall JR, Bernat EM, Patrick CJ. Externalizing psychopathology and the error-related negativity. Psychol Sci. 2007 Apr;18(4):326–33.
65 Vijayakumar N, Whittle S, Dennison M, Yücel M, Simmons J, Allen NB. Development of temperamental effortful control mediates the relationship between maturation of the prefrontal cortex and psychopathology during adolescence: a 4-year longitudinal study. Dev Cogn Neurosci. 2014 Jul;9:30–43.
66 Posner MI, Rothbart MK. Toward a physical basis of attention and self regulation. Phys Life Rev. 2009 Jun;6(2):103–20.
67 Marek S, Hwang K, Foran W, Hallquist MN, Luna B. The contribution of network organization and integration to the development of cognitive control. PLoS Biol. 2015 Dec; 13(12):e1002328.
68 Davis FC, Knodt AR, Sporns O, Lahey BB, Zald DH, Brigidi BD, et al. Impulsivity and the modular organization of resting-state neural networks. Cereb Cortex. 2013 Jun; 23(6):1444–52.
69 Menon V, Uddin LQ. Saliency, switching, attention and control: a network model of insula function. Brain Struct Funct. 2010 Jun; 214(5-6):655–67.
70 Rueter AR, Abram SV, MacDonald AW 3rd, Rustichini A, DeYoung CG. The goal priority network as a neural substrate of Conscientiousness. Hum Brain Mapp. 2018 Sep;39(9): 3574–85.
71 Farr OM, Hu S, Zhang S, Li CS. Decreased saliency processing as a neural measure of Barratt impulsivity in healthy adults. Neuroimage. 2012 Nov;63(3):1070–7.
72 Churchwell JC, Yurgelun-Todd DA. Age-related changes in insula cortical thickness and impulsivity: significance for emotional development and decision-making. Dev Cogn Neurosci. 2013 Oct;6:80–6.
73 Lewis GJ, Cox SR, Booth T, Muñoz Maniega S, Royle NA, Valdés Hernández M, et al. Trait conscientiousness and the personality meta-trait stability are associated with regional white matter microstructure. Soc Cogn Affect Neurosci. 2016 Aug;11(8):1255–61.
74 Allen TA, DeYoung CG, Bagby RM, Pollock B, Quilty LC. A hierarchical integration of normal and abnormal personality dimensions: structure and predictive validity in a heterogeneous sample of psychiatric outpatients. Assessment. 2020 Jun;27(4):643–56.
75 Watson D, Stasik SM, Ellickson-Larew S, Stanton K. Extraversion and psychopathology: A facet-level analysis. J Abnorm Psychol. 2015 May;124(2):432–46.
76 Rhodes JD, Colder CR, Trucco EM, Speidel C, Hawk LW Jr, Lengua LJ, et al. The interaction between self-regulation and motivation prospectively predicting problem behavior in adolescence. J Clin Child Adolesc Psychol. 2013; 42(5):681–92.
77 Urošević S, Collins P, Muetzel R, Schissel A, Lim KO, Luciana M. Effects of reward sensitivity and regional brain volumes on substance use initiation in adolescence. Soc Cogn Affect Neurosci. 2015 Jan;10(1):106–13.
78 Chester DS, DeWall CN. The pleasure of revenge: retaliatory aggression arises from a neural imbalance toward reward. Soc Cogn Affect Neurosci. 2016 Jul;11(7):1173–82.
79 Yang Y, Joshi SH, Jahanshad N, Thompson PM, Baker LA. Neural correlates of proactive and reactive aggression in adolescent twins. Aggress Behav. 2017 May;43(3):230–40.
80 Wright AG, Thomas KM, Hopwood CJ, Markon KE, Pincus AL, Krueger RF. The hierarchical structure of DSM-5 pathological personality traits. J Abnorm Psychol. 2012 Nov; 121(4):951–7.
81 Somerville LH, Hare T, Casey BJ. Frontostriatal Maturation Predicts Cognitive Control Failure to Appetitive Cues in Adolescents. J Cogn Neurosci. 2011 Sep;23(9):2123–34.
82 Allen TA, Rueter AR, Abram SV, Brown JS, DeYoung CG. Personality and neural correlates of mentalizing ability. Eur J Pers. 2017 Nov-Dec;31(6):599–613.
83 Rodriguez-Seijas C, Ruggero C, Eaton NR, Krueger RF. The DSM-5 alternative model for personality disorders and clinical treatment: A review. Curr Treat Options Psychiatry. 2019 Dec;6(4):284–98.
84 Milinkovic MS, Tiliopoulos N. A systematic review of the clinical utility of the DSM-5 section III alternative model of personality disorder. Personal Disord. 2020. DOI: https://doi.org/10.1037/per0000408.
85 DeYoung CG, Quilty LC, Peterson JB, Gray JR. Openness to experience, intellect, and cognitive ability. J Pers Assess. 2014;96(1): 46–52.

Review Article

Psychopathology

Psychopathology 2020;53:213–220
DOI: 10.1159/000509624

Received: March 27, 2020
Accepted: June 22, 2020
Published online: August 6, 2020

Personality Disturbances as Emergent Phenomena Reflective of Underlying Neurobehavioral Systems: Beyond Dimensional Measurement, Phenotypic Trait Descriptors, and Factor Analysis

Mark F. Lenzenweger[a–c] Richard A. Depue[d]

[a]Department of Psychology, The State University of New York at Binghamton, Binghamton, NY, USA; [b]Department of Psychiatry, Weill Cornell Medical College, New York, NY, USA; [c]Personality Disorders Institute, Weill Cornell Medical College, White Plains, NY, USA; [d]Laboratory of Neurobiology of Personality, Institute of Human Neuroscience, Department of Human Development, Cornell University, Ithaca, NY, USA

Keywords

Neurobehavioral systems · Personality disorder · Emergent phenomena · Personality neuroscience · DSM-5 Alternative Model of Personality Disorders · Personality

Abstract

Background and Overview: The conceptualization of personality pathology, or personality disturbance, is now at a substantive crossroads. Some researchers (and clinicians) prefer a focus on the domains of personality pathology that are well-described and captured in traditional categorical diagnostic approaches that, in some instances, abut normal personality constructs. Other workers argue to move the study of personality disorder (PD) closer to personality science seeking continuous connections between PD and established dimensions of healthy-range, normal personality. Most of the latter efforts revolve around correlational and factor analytic study of phenotypic expressions of PD features and normal personality dimensions. It is notable, however, that both visions of the PD/personality interface are essentially unlinked to an understanding of shared neurobiological underpinnings (i.e., neurotransmitter-influenced neurobehavioral systems) of both personality disturbance and normal personality[1]. Here, we present a nontechnical, conceptual overview of our approach to this problem, advancing a neurobehavioral approach that seeks to anchor both normal personality and personality disturbance within a matrix of brain-based neurobiological systems, incorporating genetic, epigenetic, and environmental inputs. In this brief paper, we seek only to provide a necessarily cursory introduction to how we conceptualize this area and illustrate, in broad outline, our effort to characterize both personality and personality disturbance anchored in neurobehavioral systems. Our approach, which we began developing in the middle 1990s, can be juxtaposed with the more recently proposed *DSM-5* Alternative Model of Personality Disorders as well as the well-established five-factor approach to PD.

Correspondence: E-mail correspondence concerning this article may be directed to either Mark F. Lenzenweger, PhD, mlenzen@binghamton.edu or Richard A. Depue, PhD, rad5@cornell.edu.

1 In our modeling, we focus specifically on neurotransmitter systems and related neurobehavioral processes. We do not focus on functional neuroanatomy findings from neuroimaging studies of personality disordered participants, nor do we base our modeling on neuroimaging correlates of personality dimensions (e.g., five-factor approach).

karger@karger.com
www.karger.com/psp

Karger

Mark F. Lenzenweger
Department of Psychology
State University of New York at Binghamton
Binghamton, NY 13902 (USA)
mlenzen@binghamton.edu

Domains of Inquiry Converge: Brief Review of the Challenges to Integration

Over the past 35 years, the field has seen efforts to understand clinical psychopathology constructs known as personality disorders (PDs) with personality science constructs that characterize models of normal-range personality. Prior to about 1985, these domains of constructs were quite separate in terms of both theory and empirical research [1]. Normal personality psychologists focused on dimensional trait conceptualizations, inventory development, and factor analytic studies of inventory data derived from, typically, university populations. Simultaneously, psychiatry and clinical psychology focused on the description and articulation of domains of PD that were long observed in the consulting room and conceived of categorically, but were less systematically delineated or conceptualized beyond atheoretical collections of signs and symptoms (e.g., antisocial personality, borderline pathology, narcissistic disorders, schizoid personality, and so on).

Two major foci of nearly all efforts seeking to bridge these two domains have been, importantly, to determine (a) whether the nature and breadth of normal personality constructs adequately map those thought to define the PD conceptual space and vice versa and (b) how the domains are fundamentally related (e.g., merely associated vs. genuinely continuous). From the 1980s through the early 2000s, a large empirical literature appeared that focused on the correlations that exist among normal personality constructs and PD concepts. The typical form of such studies was that a normal personality inventory and a measure of PD were administered to the same participants and the resulting associations across the two measures were described. Nearly all theoretical discussion regarding personality and PD sprung from empirical patterns discerned in these correlation matrices. Additionally, inspired in part by such data, many scholarly discussions of personality and PD during this time circled about the theme of "categories" versus "dimensions" and debated the best approach to conceptualization and measurement of PDs. Much of this work laid the foundation for what would eventually come to be known as the *DSM-5* Alternative Model of Personality Disorder (AMPD) [2], a hybrid categorical-dimensional model of PD that incorporated much of what is contained in the well-known five-factor approach to normal personality plus some additional constructs of a more pathological nature.

A conspicuous feature of much of the initial work linking normal personality and PD was its reliance on correlational results showing associations between *phenotypic* measures of PD features and personality dimensions. The normal personality dimensions under consideration were most commonly the five personality factors/traits of neuroticism, extraversion, openness to experience, conscientiousness, and agreeableness. Such correlations amongst the PD and personality measures were argued, by some, as evidence reflective of continuity between personality and PD (e.g., elevated borderline PD features were often associated with low levels of agreeableness or related facet). Such correlations derived from manifest indicators, however, could *not* definitively confirm continuity in latent or underlying structure.

Another feature of this corpus pointed to the insufficiency of extant normal personality constructs for explaining the wide range and highly dysfunctional aspects of personality pathology (e.g., paranoia, self-mutilation, severe narcissism, profound amounts of aggression and meanness, near total absence of fear, micro-psychotic episodes, extreme masochism). Many experienced psychopathologists saw the major extant normal personality dimensions as simply too coarse and lacking in both nuance and configural relations to validly capture the PD domain, facet measures of personality dimensions notwithstanding. Efforts to link personality and PD in a deeper manner have been relatively sparse. Early on, Gray [3] sought to develop a model linking underlying neurophysiological systems to normal personality. An alternative approach to linking PD to normal personality systems, building upon the insights of Gray and others, was proposed by Cloninger et al. [4]. Their personality model consists of two broad classes of subdomains falling within temperament or character. PD is seen, in this model, as largely reflective of diminished self-directedness (a putative character feature) with modifying inputs from harm-avoidance, novel-seeking, and/or reward-dependence, i.e., temperament factors.

Each of these issues (construct continuity, insufficient mapping of pathology, coarseness of construct conceptualization) remains unresolved to one degree or another today; however, the proposed *DSM-5* AMPD has begun to advance the discussion considerably. For example, through the AMPD, there has been some degree of convergence regarding the likely domains of normal personality related to personality pathology, and a common language has been proposed. That the AMPD has not been uniformly accepted is attested to by its inclusion as an "emerging model" in the *DSM-5* (Section III), whereas the official diagnostic criteria for PDs in *DSM-5* remained unchanged from the prior system (*DSM-IV-TR*). A critical aspect that remains strikingly minimally developed in this area of inquiry, for both normal personality and PD, is the underlying neurobiological influences at play in both normalcy and pathology in personality functioning. In this paper, we describe our approach to understanding personality and personality dysfunction from the standpoint of neurobehavioral systems and position it for comparison with the AMPD (see other papers in this special issue).

We present our model as an overview summary of our prior extended explications of our model of personality disturbance, personality, and neurobehavioral systems. We presented our initial neurobehavioral dimensional model of PD in 2001 [5], with subsequent revision in 2005 [6]. Our most recent model has been presented more recently in considerable detail elsewhere [7, 8]. Here, we present our model succinctly in broad descriptive terms for consideration juxtaposed with the AMPD which is described extensively in the other papers in this special issue; the interested reader can consult our prior presentations for extensive technical neurobiological detail [5–8]. Our presentation focuses on (a) personality disturbance as *emergent* phenomena, which implicitly embraces a dimensional perspective, and (b) our specific neurobehavioral perspective that underpins both personality and personality disturbance.

Personality Disturbance as Emergent Phenomena Arising from Underlying Dimensionally Structured Systems

Since 2001, we have proposed that personality pathology be regarded as an emergent phenomenon [5]. Briefly, the concept of *emergence* and resultant *emergent properties*, when they arise, speak to the development or appearance of some novel condition or phenomenon that is coherent and integrated. An emergent phenomenon cannot be explained by reference to its constituent parts or contributing components. Stated differently, the emergent entity or phenomenon along with its properties cannot be predicted from the elements that make up the entity. In short, importantly, the emergent phenomenon is *more* than the simple sum of its parts. Emergence, as a descriptive organizing concept and process, plays a critical role in many areas of science. For example, emergent processes and properties figure centrally in fields as divergent as condensed matter and material physics to animal behavior to meteorology to contemporary cognitive neuroscience. There are many common examples of emergent phenomenon, such as bird flocking, the game of chess, hurricanes, and ant colonies. In psychological science, for example, one might think of the experience of consciousness or visual imagery as emergent properties of the brain (or, more specifically, neural circuits, neurobiological systems, and structures within the brain) [e.g., 9–11]. Furthermore, one could think of "rigidity" or "contour" as emergent properties of an object without reference to the physical components that make up an object. We [5–7, 12] have argued that the concept of emergence is relevant to the psychopathology of the personality as well as most forms of disturbance represent complex configural outcomes of multiple interacting systems.

Specifically, we have argued that personality *disorders* as relatively discrete disease entities, such as conceived of within the traditional diagnostic nomenclatures, do not exist per se [6–8]. As an alternative, we proposed a perspective, where personality disturbance represents *emergent* phenotypes that arise from the interaction of extreme values on critical subsets of major personality systems, which are reflected in what are termed traits reflective of underlying neurobehavioral systems and structured dimensionally. That is, each individual's personality represents the interaction of all major underlying neurobehavioral systems. In this context, we note that the term *emergent* is used to describe personality pathology as configurations of disturbance that "emerge" or "arise" from the novel combination of constituent personality systems, but such configurations of disturbance cannot be reduced or parsed readily into those contributing neurobehavioral systems. Where individuals lie at the extreme (low or high) ends of interacting trait dimensions on subsets of the major neurobehavioral systems (which we identify phenotypically as traits), emotional behavior emerges that generates social and/or occupational impairment, rendering disturbance in the individual's life resulting from these personality systems.

This general model follows from our position that higher-order traits of personality reflect the activities of neurobehavioral systems [7, 12–17]. Though genetically speaking it may be possible to conceive of the neurobiological variables associated with neurobehavioral systems as subject to independent influences, it is impossible to imagine that these systems are independent at a functional level. Neurobehavioral systems, and the personality traits that reflect their influence, interact to produce complex behavior patterns – personality as a whole – in a multivariate, interactive fashion [see 7, 12, and below for more discussion of this issue]. Although this model is fully dimensional in nature, where personality disturbance lies at the extreme of normal, interacting personality di-

Psychopathology 2020;53:213–220
DOI: 10.1159/000509624

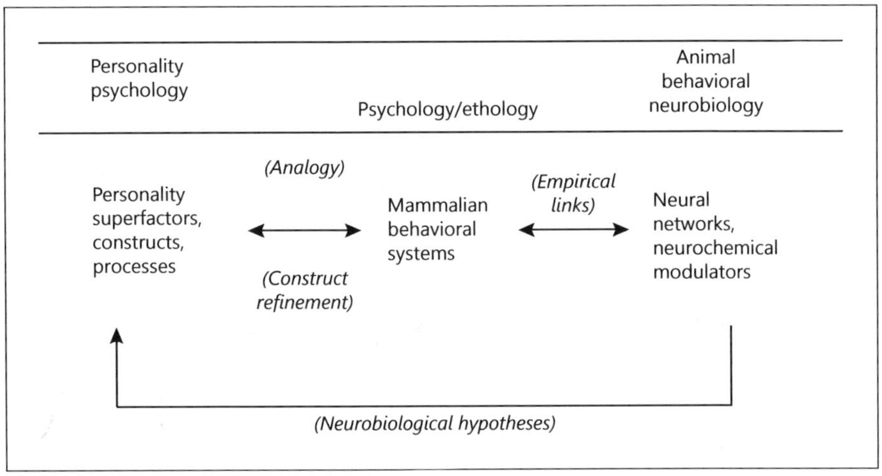

Fig. 1. A modeling strategy for deriving neurobiological hypotheses about higher-order traits of personality and personality disturbance. Copyright © 2014 by R.A. Depue and M.F. Lenzenweger. Used with permission.

mensions, no assumption is made herein that phenotypic dimensions of personality are genetically continuous. The phenotypic continuity could well represent several underlying *distinct* genotypic distributions, as may be the case even within the normal range of variation of some personality traits [13].

Conceptual Overview of a Neurobehavioral Model Underpinning Both Personality and Personality Disturbance

Before reviewing our model, we believe it is important to address a prior model of PD that embraces neurobiological determinants. It is one that views PD largely in terms of subsyndromal or preclinical expressions of liabilities for major forms of psychopathology (i.e., psychotic illness, affective disorders, and so on). Siever and colleagues [18, 19] proposed that PDs represented subsyndromal expressions of major forms of psychopathology. Borderline PD, for example, is viewed as a variant of affective disorder. Borderline PD, in Siever et al.'s approach, is viewed essentially as a subsyndromal variant of affective illness marked by affective instability as a central criterion as well as high levels of impulse dyscontrol and aggression, thus seen largely as pathological dysfunction in serotonergic functioning. Importantly, as distinguished from our model, the Siever model fails to capture the interactive nature of multiple underlying neurobiological processes that set the stage for personality pathology.

In developing our neurobehavioral model of personality disturbance, we extended the strategy originally described in Depue and Collins [14] to personality disturbance as outlined in Figure 1. Personality psychology was used to define the behavioral, emotional, and motivational characteristics of molar dimensions of normal-range human personality (e.g., extraversion). Next, we identified mammalian behavior patterns with corresponding characteristics, as described in the psychological and ethological literatures. Once an analogous motivation was identified, the animal neurobiological research was consulted, and that corpus provided empirical links to its neural organization and neurochemical modulation. These hypotheses were then extended to humans and were defined in a manner allowing for empirical tests. Once the major neurobehavioral systems were identified through this process, we sought to conceptualize well-known patterns of personality disturbance within the multidimensional space defined by these systems [5–7].

Our multidimensional model of personality disturbance is illustrated in Figure 2. In the model, the axes are defined by neurobehavioral systems [7, 8, 14–17, 20] rather than by personality traits, because traits are only approximate, fallible (phenotypic) estimates of these systems. It is also essential to note that we do not seek to place the established categorical DSM-system PDs within this multidimensional construct space. In a prior effort, we [5] demonstrated that one could approximate the location of DSM PDs in such a multidimensional space. However, our current view [7–8] is that the model allows for a richer depiction of regions of personality dysfunction depicted in the mapped *reaction surface* in Figure 2. The regions of dysfunction accord well with variation on the underlying neurobehavioral systems, would reveal themselves in phenotypic disturbance, and do not require reliance on DSM PD constructs.

Psychopathology 2020;53:213–220
DOI: 10.1159/000509624

Our model consists of multiple neurobehavioral systems: incentive motivation, anxiety/stress reactivity, affiliative reward, rejection sensitivity, neural (nonaffective) constraint, affective aggression, and fear. Furthermore, each of these neurobehavioral systems is modulated by one or more neurotransmitter systems of wide brain distribution [for reviews, see 7, 8, 12, 15, 20]. In Figure 2, two major neurobehavioral systems are modeled as a ratio of relative strength, because the opposing nature of their eliciting stimuli affects behavior in a reciprocal manner, such that the elicitation or expression of one system is influenced by the strength of the other: (1) a dopamine-facilitated system of behavioral approach based on positive incentive motivation, which is hypothesized to underlie extraversion and positive emotionality [12, 14, 16]; and (2) norepinephrine and corticotrophin-releasing hormone-modulated anxiety/stress reactivity [12, 15, 21], thought to underlie neuroticism and negative emotionality [6, 7, 12, 22].

Similarly, a *mu*-opiate and oxytocin-modulated affiliative reward dimension [17, 20, 23], representing the capacity to experience consummatory reward from social and soft-touch stimulation [20], and thought to underlie the trait of social closeness or agreeableness [17], is placed in ratio with rejection sensitivity. A ratio of these 2 systems is modeled, because they both largely influence the interpersonal domain but can have opposite effects on social bonding. Moreover, a dimension of rejection sensitivity likely provides a novel contribution to the traditional categories of dependent-, avoidant-, and borderline disturbance (all high on this dimension).

Finally, a neural constraint dimension is hypothesized to underlie the trait of constraint or conscientiousness. Through the interaction of serotonin, GABA, and norepinephrine, constraint provides inhibitory modulation of the threshold of stimulus elicitation of the other neurotransmitter systems [12, 15, 24–27]. Hence, in turn, the behavioral expressive features of the other neurobehavioral systems are also modulated by constraint. Due to the limitation of graphing more than 3 dimensions, it should be noted that the model includes one additional system/trait input that we suggest influences the manifestation of personality disturbance: the ratio of affective aggression:fear to account for a full range of antisocial behavior (particularly, high aggression:low fear). Thus, taken together, the model proposes that the interaction of multiple neurobehavioral-neurotransmitter systems underlying dimensional personality traits is necessary to account for the emergent phenotypes observed in personality disturbance.

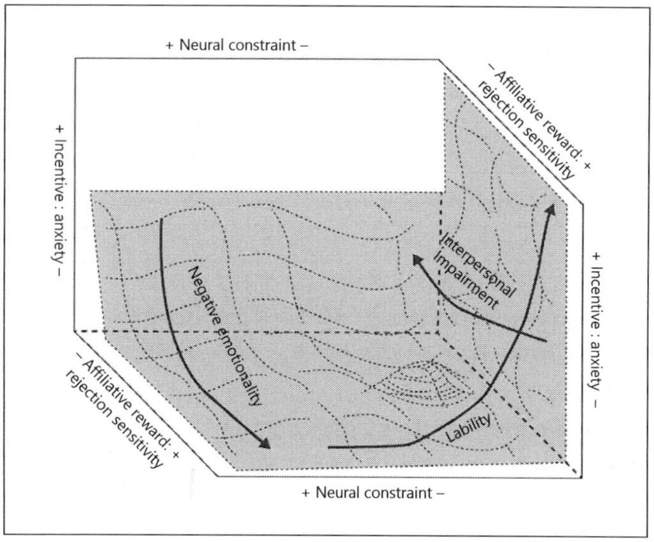

Fig. 2. A multidimensional neurobehavioral model of personality disturbance. The incentive, affiliative reward, anxiety, neural constraint, and rejection sensitivity neurobehavioral systems are depicted in terms of a reaction surface. Copyright © 2014 by R.A. Depue and M.F. Lenzenweger. Used with permission.

Three significant features of the model in Figure 2 are worth emphasizing. First, the phenotypic expression of personality disturbance, represented by the gray-shaded reaction surface in the figure (accounting for ~10% of the population [28]), is continuous in nature, changing in character gradually but seamlessly across the surface in a manner that reflects the changing product of the multidimensional interactions. Because the functioning of the neurotransmitter systems underlying neurobehavioral systems is interactive in nature, estimating the product of these multidimensional interactions most effectively is an important task for future research. One framework for such estimation was recently proposed, and it serves as an initial step in the process [12].

Second, it may be that certain areas of the reaction surface (i.e., certain system/trait interactions) are associated with increased probability (risk) of certain features of personality disturbance, perhaps having given rise initially to clinical theories of PDs based on prototypic phenotypes. An example of such increased probability is represented in the right-back area of the figure as an elevation in the surface that is continuous rather than distinct in contour. As noted above, this representation, however, is not meant to imply that a distinct disorder exists in that particular zone of the surface.

Importantly, the extent and positioning of the gray reaction surface is weighted most heavily by *increasing* anxiety/stress reactivity, *decreasing* neural constraint, and *decreasing* affiliative reward:*increasing* rejection sensitivity. This weighting is also reflected in the lines with directional arrows overlaying the gray surface in Figure 2, which illustrate increasing phenotypic negative emotionality, emotional lability, and interpersonal impairment. These three factors were found to be the most common characteristics of all PDs in a meta-analysis [29], and a study by Kendler et al. [30] showed independent genetic contributions to these factors, thereby empirically supporting their emphasis in the model.

Third, our modeling of personality disturbance accounts for the nature of dysfunction found to occur in most well-known forms of personality disturbance [2, Section I] irrespective of reliance on presumed DSM categorical structure. Importantly, in this context, we note that we have advocated for a view that both schizotypal and paranoid disturbances are less likely to be effectively modeled as variants of personality and its underlying neurobehavioral substrates. This position is informed by the substantial corpus of data that identifies these forms of psychopathology as intimately related to schizophrenia per se rather than personality. We have argued that these conditions more accurately represent alternative manifestations of the liability for schizophrenia [31, 32]. As such, we have not sought to model schizotypal and paranoid pathology within our neurobehavioral framework (in this context, we also note the AMPD posits a "psychoticism" personality factor, which we do *not* include in our framework as per our discussion of schizophrenia-related pathology).

There are other points of divergence in our model vis a vis the *DSM-5* AMPD [2, Section III]. For example, we see the positive emotion/incentive reward system as playing a critical role in the emergence of normal personality as well as personality disturbance, particularly in relation to anxiety, whereas positive emotion does not play a central role in the *DSM-5* AMPD. An expanded AMPD would need to incorporate explicitly positive emotion. We also note our explicit focus on rejection sensitivity as an important dimension/process within our proposed model, which is an important point of divergence from the AMPD. The AMPD describes "separation insecurity," but only as a sub-domain of negative emotion, which is not necessarily reflective solely of rejection sensitivity. In our modeling, we seek to avoid blended phenotypic constructs such as "impulsivity," which reflects at least five systems, such as positive incentive motivation, fear, affective and competitive aggression, and nonaffective constraint. Rather, we prefer a focus on the nature of the underlying neurobehavioral systems, which in interaction allow for the emergence of heterogenous, blended behavioral phenotypic outcomes.

Many additional implications of our model are discussed in detail elsewhere [7–8], but two seem important in the consideration of the *development* of personality disturbance. First, each of the neurotransmitters discussed above are subject to significant and long-lasting modification in functioning by early postnatal experience [12, 20]. Exactly which types of early experience are most impactful on which neurotransmitters is currently an area of intense research [20]. Nevertheless, it is clear that genetically influenced effects on neurotransmitter functioning alter human perceptual, cognitive, motor, and affective responses to environmental contexts [14, 16, 20, 23]. Thus, in this framework, elevation and dynamic movement in the reaction surface of the model could be strongly influenced by current but historically meaningful environmental contexts. Therefore, it would seem that this area of research could profitably be integrated with clinical and research accounts of personality disturbance.

Second, sex differences in some forms of personality disturbance may imply differential risk (neurobiological and/or environmental) based on biological sex and/or psychological gender-related influences. The increased prevalence of males with antisocial behavior may reflect the higher mean of males in the population on the ratio of traits of aggression:fear and a lower mean on constraint [26, 27]. Additionally, the increased prevalence of females with borderline- and dependent-like personality disturbance seen in some samples (though not all) may reflect a combination of (a) their higher mean on both trait anxiety; (b) their higher mean on social closeness, thereby increasing the need for social relationships whose loss is feared; (c) their higher mean on rejection sensitivity, thereby increasing their vacillation between dependence and rejection of others; (d) their lower mean on extraversion, particularly social dominance, hence enhancing the predominance of high levels of trait anxiety; and (e) their lower mean on the ratio of aggression:fear, hence decreasing the prevalence of antisocial behavior [7, 12, 14, 17, 33].

We see neurobiologically informed study of the development of personality disturbance, particularly as related to the appearance of sex differences, as an area ripe for future research. For example, while one could pursue numerous vectors of research, issues of particular importance are (a) how subcortical neural systems of approach and avoidance develop much sooner than cortical neural systems of self-regulation; (b) how cortical neural development is compromised in many PDs; and (c) how environmental insults can affect cortical development [34]. Inclusion of evolutionary perspectives on a neurobiologically-based model of personality and personality disturbance development could also be considered [e.g., 35]. Finally, it would be useful to seek connections among the neurobehavioral systems indicators that we discuss here and clinically relevant measures of functional impairment.

We offer this neurobehavioral perspective on the emergence of personality and personality disturbance for consideration vis a vis other personality approaches, such as the five-factor approach and the AMPD. For example, while the five-factor conceptualizations (five-factor model, Big-5) of personality and PDs maintain their traction in some quarters, the AMPD has gained a substantial foothold in the scientific study of PD since its introduction in 2013 [2]. However, what remains striking is that both the five-factor approach as well as the AMPD approach remain largely disconnected from neurobiological modeling; rather, they are anchored in the correlational and factor analytic frameworks that seek to explore the interface of personality and personality disturbance through patterns of association of phenotypic indicators. We offer our model as a heuristic and substantive explanation of the underlying nature of both personality and personality disturbance. We believe it suggests an integrated basis for understanding both personality and personality disturbance while simultaneously suggesting important vectors for empirical research across levels of analysis, ranging from the genetic and epigenetic [see 7 for extensive discussion of genetic and epigenetic considerations], through neurobiology, to neurocognitive processes [36] and phenotypic individual differences, all the while allowing for interpersonal [37] and environmental inputs.

Statement of Ethics

Ethics approval was not required for this report as it is a statement of theory.

Conflict of Interest Statement

The authors have no conflicts of interest to declare.

Funding Sources

This theory development work was supported in part by National Institute of Mental Health Research Grants MH-45448 to M.F. Lenzenweger and MH-55347 to R.A. Depue.

Author Contributions

Mark F. Lenzenweger: theory development, PDs, personality; Richard A. Depue: theory development, PDs, personality.

References

1 Widiger TA, Frances A. The DSM-III personality disorders. Perspectives from psychology. Arch Gen Psychiatry. 1985 Jun;42(6):615–23.
2 American Psychiatric Association. Diagnostic and statistical manual of mental disorders (DSM-5). 5th ed. Arlington (VA): American Psychiatric Publishing; 2013.
3 Gray JA. The psychology of fear and stress. Problems in the behavioural sciences. Volume 5. 2nd ed. Cambridge, England: Cambridge University Press; 1987.
4 Cloninger CR, Svrakic DM, Przybeck TR. A psychobiological model of temperament and character. Arch Gen Psychiatry. 1993 Dec; 50(12):975–90.
5 Depue RA, Lenzenweger MF. A neurobehavioral dimensional model of personality disorders. In: Livesley WJ, editor. The Handbook of Personality Disorders. New York: Guilford; 2001. pp. 136–76.
6 Depue RA, Lenzenweger MF. A neurobehavioral model of personality disturbance. In: Lenzenweger MF, Clarkin JF, editors. Major theories of personality disorder. 2nd ed. New York: Guilford; 2005. pp. 391–453.
7 Lenzenweger MF, Depue RA. Toward a developmental psychopathology of personality disturbance: A neurobehavioral dimensional model incorporating genetic, environmental, and epigenetic factors. In: Cicchetti D, editor. Maladaptation and Psychopathology. Developmental Psychopathology. Volume 3. 3rd ed. New York: Wiley; 2016. pp. 1079–110.
8 Depue R, Fu Y. Neurogenetic and experiential processes underlying major personality traits: implications for modelling personality disorders. Int Rev Psychiatry. 2011 Jun;23: 258–81.
9 Rumelhart DE. The emergence of cognitive phenomena from sub-symbolic processes. In: Proceedings of the Sixth Annual Conference of the Cognitive Science Society. Hillsdale, NJ: Lawrence Erlbaum; 1984. pp. 59–62.
10 Kosslyn SM, Pomerantz JR. Imagery, propositions, and the form of internal representations. Cognit Psychol. 1977;9(1):52–76.
11 McClelland JL, Botvinick MM, Noelle DC, Plaut DC, Rogers TT, Seidenberg MS, et al. Letting structure emerge: connectionist and dynamical systems approaches to cognition. Trends Cogn Sci. 2010 Aug;14(8):348–56.
12 Moore SR, Depue RA. Neurobehavioral foundation of environmental reactivity. Psychol Bull. 2016 Feb;142(2):107–64.
13 Depue RA. Interpersonal behavior and the structure of personality: Neurobehavioral foundation of agentic extraversion and affiliation. In: Canli T, editor. Biology of Personality and Individual Differences. New York: Guilford Press; 2006. pp. 60–92.
14 Depue RA, Collins PF. Neurobiology of the structure of personality: dopamine, facilitation of incentive motivation, and extraversion. Behav Brain Sci. 1999 Jun;22(3):491–517.
15 Depue RA, Fu Y. The neurobiology and neurochemistry of temperament in adults. In: Zentner M, Shiner RL, editors. The Handbook of Temperament. New York: Guilford Press; 2012. pp. 368–99.

16 Depue RA, Fu Y. On the nature of extraversion: variation in conditioned contextual activation of dopamine-facilitated affective, cognitive, and motor processes. Front Hum Neurosci. 2013 Jun;7:288.
17 Depue RA, Morrone-Strupinsky JV. A neurobehavioral model of affiliative bonding: implications for conceptualizing a human trait of affiliation. Behav Brain Sci. 2005 Jun;28(3): 313–50.
18 Siever LJ, Davis KL. A psychobiological perspective on the personality disorders. Am J Psychiatry. 1991 Dec;148(12):1647–58.
19 Siever LJ, Weinstein LN. The neurobiology of personality disorders: implications for psychoanalysis. J Am Psychoanal Assoc. 2009 Apr;57(2):361–98.
20 Fu Y, Depue RA. A novel neurobehavioral framework of the effects of positive early postnatal experience on incentive and consummatory reward sensitivity. Neurosci Biobehav Rev. 2019 Dec;107:615–40.
21 White TL, Depue RA. Differential association of traits of fear and anxiety with norepinephrine- and dark-induced pupil reactivity. J Pers Soc Psychol. 1999 Oct;77(4):863–77.
22 Canli T. Toward a neurogenetic theory of neuroticism. Ann N Y Acad Sci. 2008;1129(1): 153–74.
23 Fu Y, Selcuk E, Moore SR, Depue RA. Touch-induced face conditioning is mediated by genetic variation in opioid but not oxytocin receptors. Sci Rep. 2018;8:9004.
24 Carver CS, Miller CJ. Relations of serotonin function to personality: current views and a key methodological issue. Psychiatry Res. 2006 Sep;144(1):1–15.
25 Depue RA, Spoont MR. Conceptualizing a serotonin trait. A behavioral dimension of constraint. Ann N Y Acad Sci. 1986;487:47–62.
26 Spoont MR. Modulatory role of serotonin in neural information processing: implications for human psychopathology. Psychol Bull. 1992 Sep;112(2):330–50.
27 Zald DH, Depue RA. Serotonergic functioning correlates with positive and negative affect in psychiatrically healthy males. Pers Individ Dif. 2001 Jan;30(1):71–86.
28 Lenzenweger MF, Lane MC, Loranger AW, Kessler RC. DSM-IV personality disorders in the National Comorbidity Survey Replication. Biol Psychiatry. 2007 Sep;62(6):553–64.
29 Saulsman LM, Page AC. The five-factor model and personality disorder empirical literature: A meta-analytic review. Clin Psychol Rev. 2004 Jan;23(8):1055–85.
30 Kendler KS, Aggen SH, Czajkowski N, Røysamb E, Tambs K, Torgersen S, et al. The structure of genetic and environmental risk factors for DSM-IV personality disorders: a multivariate twin study. Arch Gen Psychiatry. 2008 Dec;65(12):1438–46.
31 Lenzenweger MF. Schizotypy and schizotypic psychopathology: Mapping an alternative expression of schizophrenia liability. In: Lenzenweger MF, Dworkin RH, editors. Origins and development of schizophrenia: Advances in experimental psychopathology. Washington (DC): American Psychological Association; 1998. pp. 93–121.
32 Lenzenweger MF. Schizotypy and schizophrenia: The view from experimental psychopathology. New York: Guilford Press; 2010. ISBN 978-1-60623-865-3.
33 Tellegen A, Waller NG. Exploring personality through test construction: development of the Multidimensional Personality Questionnaire. In: Boyle GJ, Matthews G, Saklofske DH, editors. The SAGE handbook of personality theory and assessment, Vol. 2. Personality measurement and testing. London, England: Sage Publications; 2008. pp. 261–292.
34 Beauchaine TP. A developmental psychopathology perspective on the emergence of antisocial and borderline personality pathologies across the lifespan: commentary on personality pathology in youth. In: Lejuez CW, Gratz KL, editors. The Cambridge handbook of personality disorders. New York, NY: Cambridge University Press; 2020. pp. 94–98.
35 Panksepp J. Affective neuroscience: The foundations of human and animal emotions. Oxford, England: Oxford University Press; 1998.
36 Lenzenweger MF, Clarkin JF, Fertuck EA, Kernberg OF. Executive neurocognitive functioning and neurobehavioral systems indicators in borderline personality disorder: a preliminary study. J Pers Disord. 2004 Oct;18(5): 421–38.
37 Savage M, Lenzenweger MF. The impact of social exclusion on “Reading the Mind in the Eyes” performance in relation to borderline personality disorder features. J Pers Disord. 2018 Feb;32(1):109–30.

Author Index Vol. 53, No. 3–4, 2020

karger@karger.com
www.karger.com/psp

Karger

Psychopathology

Subject Index Vol. 53, No. 3–4, 2020

karger@karger.com
www.karger.com/psp

Karger